SIMPLE STEPS

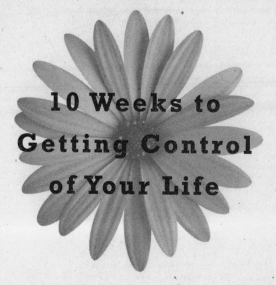

10 Weeks to Getting Control of Your Life

Health ✦ Weight ✦ Home ✦ Spirit

Lisa Lelas

Linda McClintock

Beverly Zingarella

NEW AMERICAN LIBRARY

New American Library
Published by New American Library, a division of
Penguin Putnam Inc., 375 Hudson Street, New York, New York 10014, U.S.A.
Penguin Books Ltd, 80 Strand, London WC2R 0RL, England
Penguin Books, Australia Ltd, 250 Camberwell Road, Camberwell, Victoria 3124, Australia
Penguin Books Canada Ltd, 10 Alcorn Avenue, Toronto, Ontario, Canada M4V 3B2
Penguin Books, (N.Z.) Ltd, Cnr Rosedale and Airborne Roads, Albany, Auckland 1310, New Zealand

Penguin Books Ltd, Registered Offices:
Harmondsworth, Middlesex, England

First published by New American Library, a division of Penguin Putnam Inc.

First Printing, May 2003

10   9   8   7   6   5   4   3   2   1

 REGISTERED TRADEMARK—MARCA REGISTRADA

LIBRARY OF CONGRESS CATALOGING-IN-PUBLICATION DATA

Lelas, Lisa.
Simple steps : 10 weeks to getting control of your life /
Lisa Lelas, Linda McClintock; and Beverly Zingarella.
p.   cm.
Includes bibliographical references and index.
ISBN 0-451-20862-5 (alk. paper)
1. Women—health and hygiene.   2. Women—Conduct of life.
I. McClintock, Linda.   II. Zingarella, Beverly.   III. Title.

RA778 .L536 2003
613'.04244—dc21   2002040956

Printed in the United States of America

Set in Filosofia
Designed by Jennifer Ann Daddio

To John, Lindsay, and Lexy,
who light up my life with simple joy.
—LL

To Duncan and Michael,
who capture the spirit of my soul.
—LM

To Tom, Alicia, Matthew, and Lucian,
who warm my heart with unconditional love.
—BZ

Acknowledgments

First we would like to thank author Cheryl Richardson for the Oprah connection and Cynthia Goldberg for her interest in our story. Thank you to Oprah for believing in the power of women's groups and inspiring all women to live their best life.

We would like to acknowledge our hometown newspaper, the *Shore Line Times*, of Guilford, Connecticut, for publishing the very first story about us. You were the gentle breeze before the storm.

Thank you to Lu Ann Cahn for giving us the boost to get started already and for her contributions to the interviews. Thank you to our agent, Carol Mann, for pointing us in the right direction, to Marjory Garrison, for always keeping us on track, and to our editor, Claire Zion, for believing in our passion.

Thank you to our original focus group ladies and all our Simple Steps participants for believing in us and loving the program as much as we do.

And, of course, special thanks to our families, for all of their unconditional love and support. Thank you, Alicia, for playing camp counselor to the little ones, giving us the writing time we needed.

Contents

Preface   ix

Beginnings: The Seeds Are Planted . . .   1

Getting Started: Buds to Blossoms   9

Week One: The Water Lily   17

Water · Walk · Drawers, Cabinets, and Closets · Money

Week Two: The Daisy   51

Food Journaling · Isometrics · Laundry · Daily Planning

Week Three: The Rose   77

Vitamins · Posture and Breathing · Desktop · Cleansing Routine

Week Four: The Buttercup   105

*Good Fats · Kitchen Dancing · Refrigerator and Pantry ·
Dental Hygiene*

Week Five: Lavender   133

Caffeine Cutback · Yoga · Mail Clutter · Daily Serenity Time

Week Six: The Tulip 161

Trading Carbs · Crunches · A Clean Car · Dressing Smart

Week Seven: The Morning Glory 187

Honoring Food · Stretching · Organizing Photos · Gratitude Journal

Week Eight: The Evening Primrose 215

No Night Eating · Strength Training · Your Bed · Sleep

Week Nine: The Pansy 241

Spice Up Your Life · Cross-training · Fix It · Passions

Week Ten: The Sunflower 269

Grocery Shopping · Add More Walking · Entryway · Treasure Mapping

The Harvest: Reaping the Benefits 295

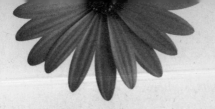

Preface

I've been a television reporter for twenty-five years. I covered the September 11th terrorist attack in New York. I was in Waco for the Davidian cult standoff. I reported from the Atlanta Olympics in the midst of the bombing and from Israel after attacks on civilians. I've met presidents, entertainment stars, felons, and scoundrels, and I believe I've seen some of the best and the worst the human spirit has to offer. I'm also a wife, a mother, and a breast cancer survivor. With that said, there are few things that surprise me anymore.

Still, every once in a rare while, in all this turmoil and tumult, you come across a story that is so honest and true it makes you reevaluate yourself and the way you live—something that speaks to your soul and helps to instruct you on how to live in this chaotic and stressful world. That's what happened when I was introduced to Simple Steps.

I met the creators of Simple Steps two years ago on assignment for NBC 10 NEWS in Philadelphia. I took a train with a photographer to meet three women in Guilford, Connecticut, who, I was told, had designed a self-improvement program that was changing women's lives. I was skeptical but agreed to go look at it. I was engaged by the creative passion and wisdom of the "Guilford Girls." Linda, Bev, and Lisa showed me their ten-week, forty-step program, and it immediately made sense to me. I knew they'd put their finger on the things that we all need to feel good about and that put us in control of our lives and our bodies. I also knew they had success stories that would inspire women everywhere to realize their potential.

In February 2000, we ran the first story about Simple Steps on NBC 10. After the story aired, 2,100 women logged on to our Web site, wondering how they could get the book. At that time, the book was just a dream for the girls from Guilford. It's been a privilege helping to make their dream a reality, contributing to their writing and serving as a kind of muse and adviser.

I hope that you will enjoy and grow during your journey as I have, taking each Simple Step to a happier and healthier life.

—Lu Ann Cahn

BEGINNINGS

The Seeds Are Planted...

Nourished by the sun.
A time for change. New beginnings.

THE SIMPLE STEPS PROGRAM IS BORN

The Beginning

Our Story

We are not doctors. We are not celebrities. We are women just like you. Women who simply want to get their own lives in shape, feel happier, have more energy, get organized, and find balance.

Our story begins the day we looked up and realized the three of us were suddenly older, married, at home, and with children. It wasn't that we were not happy. We each cherished our home and family, but we also felt we had somehow lost ourselves. We tried to pinpoint the reasons. Was it the extra pounds that crept on? Switching from career women to stay-at-home moms? Never having enough time? For each of us, various elements were different, but we all agreed that we needed a change. We had to develop more productive routines, get organized, and start putting ourselves at the top of our priority lists. We knew in our hearts that once we got our *lives* into shape, our bodies would follow, not the other way around.

We walked together. That's how our Simple Steps journey evolved. We all loved to walk . . . and talk! Lisa and Beverly, living across the street from each other on a quiet wooded hill, would steal away from sleeping families in the early morning hours to walk.

Lisa's sister, Linda, had just moved into town a few miles north, but would join in whenever she could. It became our time together.

We chatted about everything from news events to our children and husbands. We started sharing dreams and goals. We had all gained some weight after having our children, and it seemed that the talk would always turn to how we could lose it.

We didn't realize it then, but those first walks would become our first steps toward our true selves. We confided in one another. We talked about our true passions and interests in life, about why we couldn't take the weight off, about why we teach our children to properly care for themselves but don't always practice what we preach. We counted on one another. We started brainstorming about things we could do to make a difference.

One day, we met on Lisa's back deck and began to write it all down. Some of our kids were napping, others running around in the backyard, while we put pen to paper and gave solid form to the ideas we had discussed.

That was the lightbulb moment. We started to create a simple lifestyle plan. We built it out of baby steps, beginning with all the healthy tips we gave our children. We decided the best way to take our baby steps was slowly, working them into our daily routines one week at a time. We knew it takes three to four weeks to make a habit your own and we wanted lots of new, healthy habits, so we knew our plan would take time.

We started scheduling regular meetings once or twice a week, in Bev's kitchen, on Lisa's deck, or in Linda's living room. We had countless meetings that summer, took scores of notes, and did careful research, and finally we came up with a plan. *We needed to begin focusing on specific goals, such as moving more, eating healthier, and establishing efficient routines, in order to take control of our lives.*

The three of us eagerly and enthusiastically gave our own personal gifts to the program: Linda, a nutritionist by hobby, gave us healthy food perspectives. Beverly, with her strong willpower, shared tips and secrets for successful dieting and exercise. Lisa, a personal life coach and writer, developed the de-cluttering ideas and put our thoughts into words. Together we researched and created our first director's manual.

In the end, we had a simple lifestyle plan made up of forty baby steps to be performed in ten weeks. The plan encompassed everything we needed to live a better, happier, and healthier life.

The Simple Steps program looked too good not to share with other women. But would they join in? It was time to find out.

We posted flyers throughout our Connecticut shoreline community in grocery stores, libraries, community centers, and churches, but the phone did not ring. For a fleeting moment, it looked as though we developed the Simple Steps program for us . . . and just for us. Then our local newspaper called. One of the reporters had noticed a flyer and thought it might make a nice story. Well, the story was almost a full page, and as a result, our phones began ringing off the hook. So many woman—career women, stay-at-home moms, seniors, empty nesters, cancer survivors, and retirees—wanted to take part in our proposed focus group to try out the program that we could not accommodate them all. We selected twenty-three women of various backgrounds and ages to start with.

We formed a morning group and an evening group, each of which met once a week. We used our director's manual as a guide, sharing healthy living and organizational tips, and gave out four Simple Step assignments each week for the group to practice. After just a couple of weeks, we were all not only becoming good friends, but were living proof that the program was working: We were de-stressing, reorganizing, planning goals, making time for passions, pampering ourselves, eating better, moving more, saving money, getting happier, and many of us were losing weight.

The women in that first group lost a total of 300 pounds in ten weeks. But their successes surpassed simple weight losses. Some women managed to quit smoking; others rediscovered their passions and started their own businesses. One woman swears her marriage was saved by her new attitude. They were all happier and healthier.

Quite amazingly, during that very first workshop, we got a call from a producer at *The Oprah Winfrey Show* in Chicago. We didn't know it then, but our little Simple Steps program (at the time called Reflections) was about to take a giant leap! Not only did we appear on *Oprah*, but we were covered by NBC affiliate news programs across the country and countless other media outlets. We were spinning from all the publicity. We were making appearances and doing guest lectures, setting up new workshops for more and more women, and training new facilitators to help run the programs. Less than six months after creating our first focus group, we had franchised groups all around the country. Just before our one-year anniversary, we decided to write this book.

At the very first Simple Steps focus group meeting, we had kidded around that if we did well, maybe we could make it onto *The Oprah Winfrey Show*. "It was our carrot!" says Kara, one of the group's members. Indeed it was. Chasing that carrot had been inspirational fuel for all of us. Never in our wildest dreams had we expected that exactly three weeks from that first day, *The Oprah Winfrey Show* would call. Be careful what you wish for—you just might get it!

About the Authors

Lisa Lelas is a freelance writer, part-time drama teacher, and personal life coach. She facilitates many of the Simple Steps group programs in her community and across the country. She writes a newspaper column called "Life Styling with Lisa." As a public speaker, Lisa counsels that all goals are achievable by focusing on passions, following dreams with positive energy and hard work, and having a clear life plan in place. She and her husband, John, live in the quiet seaside town of Guilford, Connecticut, with their two daughters Lindsay and Lexy, and their Maltese puppy, Daisy.

Lisa loves drawing and painting, scrapbooking, doing crafts with her kids, traveling to exotic places, and gardening, and she has rekindled her passion for writing children's books. An organizer by nature, she enjoys maintaining many of the Simple Steps, especially clearing drawers and cabinets. A consummate list maker, Lisa also keeps a gratitude journal, drinks her water, walks every day, and makes a point to find some serenity time on a daily basis.

Linda McClintock, corporate MBA recruiter turned full-time mom and a nutritionist by hobby, tests and creates recipes for the workshop, provides help and information about nutrition to the participants, and keeps the books for Simple Steps. Her knowledge and research of healthy eating and living provides many of the basic principles for the Simple Steps program. She and her husband, Duncan, live in Guilford, Connecticut, with their young son, Michael, and their kitty cat, Tiger Lily.

Linda has gotten back to her passions of gourmet cooking, cake decorating, and designing and making jewelry. She also enjoys working out at the gym, gardening, entertaining, white-water rafting, and vacationing. Her favorite Simple Steps include yoga, food journaling, cross-training, trading carbs or fats, using herbs and spices in new recipes, and meal planning. Her son loves to kitchen dance with his mom.

Beverly Zingarella is a full-time mom. She facilitates local and national Simple Steps group programs. Beverly finds it rewarding to motivate other women to live their healthiest, best life. She and her husband, Tom, live in Guilford, Connecticut, with their three children, Alicia, Matthew, and Lucian, along with Ivory the cat and Labrador puppies Lilly and Bregro.

Beverly is passionate about physical activity and loves racewalking, yoga, hiking, and bicycle riding. Maintaining an orderly house keeps life in control for Bev. Some of her favorite Simple Steps include drinking lots of water daily, practicing yoga, and being aware of her posture and breathing. Drinking water, walking, and not eating after eight p.m. were the keys to Bev's weight loss and now maintain her healthy lifestyle. Finding serenity time and creating her treasure map are two Simple Steps that help Bev look forward to the future.

GETTING STARTED

Buds
to
Blossoms

Ready to open. Eager to grow.
Peeking into new horizons.

PREPARING TO BEGIN YOUR
SIMPLE STEPS JOURNEY

Getting Started

Preparing to Begin Your
Simple Steps Journey

"A journey of a thousand miles must begin with a single step."
—CHINESE PROVERB

Welcome to the Simple Steps program. Get ready to embark on a unique week-by-week approach to daily living based on simple commonsense changes.

The key to success on this journey is self-acceptance. You have to start by accepting who you are right now. Begin by looking at yourself in a full-length mirror and giving yourself a compliment out loud. Go ahead and do it. Start sending positive messages to your mind, and remember that we become who we believe we are.

In order to receive the greatest benefit from this program, you must commit the next ten weeks to making healthy changes. Read one chapter each week and follow the guidelines suggested. Make it a priority, a promise to yourself, and everything else will fall into place.

The Basic Concept

The first week, you will be assigned four Simple Steps to incorporate into your daily life. Each following week, four new steps will be added and woven into your lifestyle. Simple Steps assignments are drawn from the following four categories:

- **Health:** Nutritional awareness. Learning to make healthier food choices.
- **Weight:** Taking control of your weight through a range of activities designed for women of all fitness levels.
- **Home:** Gain control of your surroundings by de-cluttering and setting up efficient organizational systems.
- **Spirit:** Take care of yourself with fun and healthy routines.

To maximize the potential benefits of the program, we recommend that you compound each of the Simple Steps week after week. In other words, add week two's steps to your routine while continuing to practice the steps from week one, and so on. It is said that twenty-eight days of practicing change can make a new habit. The Simple Steps approach is based on this basic principle. The purpose of the Simple Steps program is to create many new healthy lifestyle habits . . . for the rest of your life.

At the end of each chapter we share some of the real-life stories of women who have found success through the Simple Steps program: success through weight loss, stress reduction, healthier cooking, home organization, and more. Let the stories inspire you. They prove that simple changes can lead to magnificent results.

How you venture into the Simple Steps journey is up to you. What you put into this, you will take out. We have found, however, that success comes easier for some when they have connections to others with similar goals. Changes are often easier to face with positive support.

1. If you choose to take this journey alone, use this book as your weekly guide and make sure to give yourself positive reinforcement daily.
2. If you want to do this with a support group, gather your own support from friends and family, or organize a Simple Steps

lifestyle makeover group in your community. Schedule weekly meetings and use this book as your text to inspire discussion. Support group kits are available, if needed.

3. If you would like on-line support, visit our Web site to discuss your program with others practicing Simple Steps. Our Web site address is www.SimpleStepsProgram.com.

The program will work for you however you choose to approach it.

Healthy Guidelines to Follow As You Begin the Program

· When starting any new dietary or exercise program, you should check with your doctor first.

· If you need to lose weight, lose at a sensible rate of ½–2 pounds per week. Keep your weight at a healthy Body Mass Index (BMI) level.

· BMI is a measure of weight in relation to height. A healthy adult BMI is considered 18.5–24.9. Anything over 29.9 is considered obese. The higher your BMI, the greater your health risks for heart disease, some cancers, breathing problems, arthritis, diabetes, and more. To find out what your BMI is, check the chart on page 14 or use this formula: Take your weight in pounds and divide it by your height in inches times itself (squared). Then take that number and multiply it by 703. For example, if you are 150 pounds and 65 inches (5 feet/5 inches), your formula is $150 \div 4,225 = .0355 \times 703 = $ BMI of 24.96.

· Eat smart, which means don't skip breakfast. It's your most important meal of the day. You need it to keep your energy level at a constant rate.

BODY MASS INDEX—YOUR BODY'S PERCENTAGE OF FAT

Weight in Pounds

Height in Feet and Inches	120	130	140	150	160	170	180	190	200	210	220	230	240	250
4'6	29	33	34	36	39	41	43	46	48	51	53	56	58	60
4'8	27	29	31	34	36	38	40	43	45	47	49	52	54	56
4'10	25	27	29	31	34	36	38	40	42	44	46	48	50	52
5'0	23	25	27	29	31	33	35	37	39	41	43	45	47	49
5'2	22	24	26	27	29	31	33	35	37	38	40	42	44	46
5'4	21	22	24	26	28	29	31	33	34	36	38	40	41	43
5'6	19	21	23	24	26	27	29	31	32	34	36	37	39	40
5'8	18	20	21	23	24	26	27	29	30	32	34	35	37	38
5'10	17	19	20	22	23	24	26	27	29	30	32	33	35	36
6'0	16	18	19	20	22	23	24	26	27	28	30	31	33	34
6'2	15	17	18	19	21	22	23	24	26	27	28	30	31	32
6'4	15	16	17	18	20	21	22	23	24	26	27	28	29	30
6'6	14	15	16	17	19	20	21	22	23	24	25	27	28	29
6'8	13	14	15	17	18	19	20	21	22	23	24	25	26	28

Healthy Weight   **Overweight**   **Obese**

From the surgeon general

FOOD PYRAMID

Let the food pyramid guide you through a healthy, balanced diet.

- **Whole Grains:** Avoid refined carbohydrates when choosing breads, cereals, rice, and pastas. Whole grains keep your energy at a steady level all day. One serving equals one slice of bread, ½ cup cooked rice or pasta, 4–6 low-fat crackers, ½ cup cooked cereal, or 1 ounce cold cereal. Eat 6–11 servings a day. For weight loss, keep it at 6.
- **Fruits:** Fruits are packed with vitamins, minerals, and cancer-fighting antioxidants. One serving equals one piece of whole fruit or 1 cup of berries or fruit chunks. Eat 2–4 servings a day.
- **Vegetables:** They're delicious and packed with vitamins, minerals, and antioxidants. One serving equals ½ cup cooked/raw or 1 cup leafy. Eat 3–5 servings a day.
- **Protein:** Meats, poultry, fish, tofu, dried beans, eggs, and nuts build and repair cells in our bodies. Eat 2–3 servings to total 4–9 ounces of cooked dried beans and peas, tofu, lean meats, poultry without skin, fish and shellfish, and eggs (preferably egg whites).
- **Dairy:** Milk, cheese, and yogurt provide calcium that is crucial to help us fight osteoporosis. One serving equals 1 cup of milk or yogurt, 1 ounce of cheese, or ½ cup soft cheese (cottage/ricotta). Eat 2–3 servings a day. If you prefer not to eat dairy, be sure to eat calcium-rich foods such as soy milk and tofu.
- **Fats and Sweets:** Eat sparingly. Less than 2 tablespoons of fats daily is enough. Limit sugar intake to as little as possible.

BEING PORTION SAVVY

- Draw an imaginary line through your plate; one half of your plate should be filled with vegetables and fruits. Divide the

other half of your plate into two equal sections, one section for
protein and the other section for whole grains.

- *Tennis ball:* the size of one serving of fruit, one serving of pasta
  or rice, two servings of a muffin, or two servings of a bagel.
- *Deck of cards:* 3-ounce serving of meat, seafood, or poultry.
- *English muffin:* 4-ounce serving of hamburger.
- *Cassette tape:* 4-ounce serving of fish.
- *CD:* One serving of a pancake.
- *Nine-volt battery:* 1 ounce of cheese.

EATING THE PROPER AMOUNTS OF FOOD

- Basing its guidelines on 2,000 calories a day, the U.S. Food and
  Drug Administration recommends that your diet should consist
  of no more than 65 grams of fat, 20 grams of saturated fat, 300
  milligrams of cholesterol, and 2,400 milligrams of sodium, and
  should include approximately 50 grams of protein, 300 grams
  of carbohydrates, 25 grams of fiber, and 3,500 milligrams of
  potassium.

The Water Lily

Simple and pure. Free-floating.
Drawing life from the earth's water gardens.

Water

Drink Eight Cups of Water Every Day

Why Do We Need Water?

- Our bodies are composed of 70 percent water and our blood is 94 percent water. Water surrounds and protects our cells, hydrates our tissue, and cleanses the wastes from our system.
- Water acts as a lubricant and cushion for our joints as well as our eyes and spinal cord.
- If your body is dehydrated, your blood becomes thicker and harder to pump, which could lead to hypertension and heart disease.
- Water acts as a coolant for our body. Water regulates a healthy body temperature, which is one reason why we sweat when we get hot.
- Our skin glows with proper hydration.
- Water washes medications from the liver.
- Water fights fatigue and gives us more energy. Without water our body cannot break down triglycerides (visualize lard) into usable forms of energy.
- Drinking a sufficient amount of water (eight cups a day) makes our metabolism burn 3 percent faster.

- Water empties stubborn fat storage deposits. Water actually carries fat out of our body.
- Water gives us a full feeling, curbing our appetite.
- By replacing one cup of regular soda a day with water, we can lose up to 10 pounds a year effortlessly.

How to Drink More Water

- This is an easy step to turn into a habit because the more water you drink, the more water your body will naturally crave.
- First, go ahead and pull out a favorite glass. Maybe a long-stem crystal glass from your china cabinet, or perhaps just a pretty glass or mug. Consider this your water glass and let it serve as a reminder to drink up.
- Drink slowly and throughout the day. If you drink your daily water requirement all at once, your body will not be able to absorb it, and it will go right through your system.
- Do not substitute other kinds of fluids for your eight glasses of water. Many drinks are dehydrating or loaded with calories.
- If you are not used to drinking water, start with four cups a day and gradually work up to the required eight by the end of the week.
- Every time you drink a beverage containing caffeine or alcohol, you should drink one to two extra glasses of water. (Caffeine and alcohol dehydrate us.)
- During aerobic workouts, remember to drink an extra cup of water every fifteen to twenty minutes.
- For weight loss, we should drink four cups of water daily for every 50 pounds we weigh. For example, if we weigh 150 pounds, we should drink twelve cups of water every day.

- Eat water-packed foods, such as melons, grapefruit, and broccoli, throughout the day.
- Easy-to-drink 8-ounce water bottles are readily available in your local grocer for those intimidated by the oversize sports bottles.
- Add a twist of lemon, lime, or orange, or a favorite fresh herb sprig for flavor.
- If you need to see color in your water, add a tablespoon or two of cranberry juice.
- Try a crunchy iced water bottle. Put a not-quite-full bottle of water in the freezer for two hours. It makes a nice treat for a warm day.
- If you like your water cold, reserve an entire shelf in your refrigerator for water so it's easy for you to grab a bottle and go.

CHATTER TIME

Don't be disheartened by the number of trips you'll make to the bathroom during your first week of drinking eight cups of water a day. Your body will soon adjust to its newly hydrated state. Kara, one of our original focus group participants, had us all chuckling when the group was asked how their first week on the program went. As her answer, she pulled out a roll of bathroom tissue from her bag and explained that this summed up her week! She had not been a water drinker previously, and until her body adjusted to it, she was forced to find every public bathroom in town.

- If you prefer room temperature water, try keeping bottles of water within reach throughout the house such as on your night-stand, desktop, and elsewhere.
- Gain support from friends and family by turning them on to the benefits and joy of water drinking.

The Key: Attaching This Step to Your Current Lifestyle

- When you wake up in the morning, make a habit of drinking your first glass of water.
- Drink a glass of water before every meal.
- Make it a point to drink an entire bottle of water while commuting to work or getting your kids to school.
- Consume another bottle of water on your commute home.
- While grocery shopping, aim for finishing a bottle of water before you check out. You will notice many of the new shopping carts now have drink holders built in for your convenience. Don't forget to pay for your water!
- Celebrate the end of the day by having a water toast with your family at the dinner table. Celebrate with loved ones that you have started your Simple Steps journey to healthier living.
- If you find your own unique way to attach this step to your personal lifestyle, please share your ideas with us on our Web site: www.SimpleStepsProgram.com.

MORE CHATTER

Jane, a Simple Steps participant, took pleasure in drinking her water out of a long-stem wineglass during the ten-week program. It was a fun way to pamper herself inexpensively! She often added ice cubes or lemon slices, or sipped out of a fancy straw, to spice it up. In between her water breaks, she got into the habit of placing her glass high up on her dining hutch so her grandchildren wouldn't knock it over. During her fifth week on the program, Jane's husband came home from work, stared at the wineglass, and quietly asked, "Honey, are you having midday parties that I don't know about?"

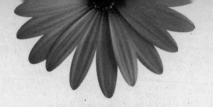

Walk

Take a Twenty-Minute Brisk Walk Every Day

Why Do We Need To Walk?

- Did you know 60 percent of Americans do not engage in regular physical activity each day? Walking is the simplest, cheapest, and most convenient way to exercise. It does not require any special equipment, other than a good pair of walking shoes. Walking can be done by people of all ages, at every fitness level.
- Walking is one of the safest forms of exercise. It is much easier on the knees and joints than running. If your pace is brisk enough (between three to four miles per hour), walking provides the same benefits as more intense aerobic activities.
- Walking strengthens our cardiovascular system and can boost the production of HDL cholesterol (the good kind) in our blood.
- A brisk walk appears to be most beneficial for most walkers. Women who said they covered one mile in fifteen to twenty minutes—an average-to-slightly-brisk pace in which one could carry on a conversation but would rather not—were also protected from cardiovascular disease according to a report in *The New England Journal of Medicine* dated September 2002.

- Walking with proper posture can ease lower back pain. It also strengthens our ankles and our abs, and improves both our equilibrium and our coordination.
- Walking lowers anxiety. This easy exercise provides an outlet for tension and nervous energy, reducing stress. Breathing in fresh oxygen and being exposed to daylight is calming and increases energy.
- Walking can actually keep us happy, according to Duke University Medical Center psychologist James Blumenthal. His November 2000 study noted that walking increases the levels of the important brain chemicals serotonin and norepinephrine, which are both actively stimulated by antidepression medication.
- Frank Perna, Ph.D., of Boston University School of Medicine, indicated in a 2002 study that these exercise-induced brain chemicals actually help us achieve the cerebral clarity that allows our emotional distractions to disappear. After all, it's hard to think clearly when you are burdened with a cluttered mind. Creative mental breakthroughs (new ideas, personal decisions, etc.) are abundant during walks.
- A brisk walk today will help us sleep better tonight.
- Walking boosts our energy. Even as little as ten minutes of daily walking can banish fatigue and increase stamina. A brisk walk in the morning raises our metabolism for the entire day.
- Walking burns more calories then jogging. In a study conducted by exercise physiologist, Wendy Kohrt, Ph.D., at Washington University in St. Louis, women walked a twelve-minute mile and then jogged a twelve-minute mile. Surprisingly, it was the walking that burned 4 percent more calories. The reason, says Kohrt, is that walking at the brisk pace requires more energy to stay grounded; jogging at the same pace is actually more efficient and thus uses less energy—hence it burns fewer calories.

- Even a nonaerobically paced walk burns approximately 125 calories in one half hour (approximately 85 calories in twenty minutes). Brisk walking burns more.
- Walking just feels good. Have fun, look around you, and enjoy the view. Every day that we walk is a beautiful day.

How to Take Your Daily Brisk Walk

THE BASICS

- Starting a twenty-minute-daily-walk plan is simple: Go out your front door and walk, at your own pace, in any direction for ten minutes. Then turn around and come back. Congratulations, you are already done with your required exercise for the day.
- If you find twenty minutes too challenging, start with ten or fifteen minutes of daily walking and work up to twenty minutes over the next week or so.
- Start at your own pace and work up to fifteen minutes per mile: Thirty-two steps in fifteen seconds is equivalent to four miles per hour, or the fifteen-minute mile. To enjoy the full health benefits of walking, you want to work up to a twelve-minute mile or five miles per hour.
- If you are new to walking, start on a flat road or on a track.
- If you are a regular walker, why not add some hilly terrain to your walk now? Adding hills to your daily walk will burn an additional 2 calories per minute. Walking with trekking poles (like cross-country ski poles) will burn about 33 percent more calories than walking without them.
- Your major muscles have memory, so vary your walking route from flat to hilly terrain, thereby working different muscles every day.

- For extreme-weather days that keep you indoors, rent one of the many new walking videos, such as Leslie Sansone's *Miracle Mile* and Denise Austin's *TrimWalk*.

EQUIPMENT

- Your feet bear your weight when you walk, so you should invest in a good pair of walking shoes. They should be flexible at the toe and rounded at the heel for smooth heel-to-toe motion. A good walking shoe should also provide side-to-side stability and have cushioning in the middle, as well as a flexible nonskid sole and a low back tab. Whether or not you have a high instep, low arches, or an uneven tread, you should bring in your old sneakers to a reputable store for evaluation, and the salesperson should be able to look at the bottom of your sneaker to see where the wear is. After explaining any foot problems you have, he or she should be able to help you find a proper shoe. Make sure that your shoes are comfortable before you walk out the door, as you don't want any blisters popping up. If you buy your sneakers on-line, note that the Web sites of many of the better sneaker companies, such as www.newbalance.com and www.reebok.com, have a guide to help you find the right fit for your foot.
- Runners land on their heels, which is why running shoes have more cushioning in the back. Walking shoes need to be wider in the front to allow feet to spread, since walkers spend more time with their entire foot on the ground.
- Heavier walkers may need to buy sturdier shoes with extra cushioning to protect bones.
- Once you log five hundred miles (about every three to six months), you should trade in your old walking shoes for a new pair.

- For evening walking, wear light-colored clothes, and a reflective vest, and remember your flashlight.
- For winter walking, wear layers and don't forget your hat. Approximately 30 percent of body heat is lost through your head.

YOUR WALK

- Always be sure to stretch out your legs before and after your walk. Muscles that get stronger will also get tighter unless you stretch them out. Facing the stairs, stand on a step and hang one of your heels off the step. Slowly push your heel down and feel the stretch throughout that leg, hold for twenty to thirty seconds, then switch to the next leg.
- During your walks, focus on being healthy, not just on tallying the miles.
- Bend your arms at a 90-degree angle and move them while you walk to help get your heart rate up.
- Walk tall and keep good posture. Shoulders should be relaxed. Keep your chin up and contract your stomach muscles to flatten your lower back. Push off with your toes and land on your heels.
- Take small but fast steps for a better workout and to reduce your chance of injury.
- Swing into walking rhythm. Bring a small radio or Walkman with earphones. Music is an excellent motivator.
- Try spurts of speed walking between telephone poles or mailboxes. This increases your calorie burn by 8–13 percent.
- Try walking backward as a great way to increase your strength and agility while keeping injuries at bay.
- If you become winded while walking briskly, reduce your speed and catch your breath. Slow to a pace that allows you to breathe deeply. You should feel able to talk, but not want to carry on a conversation.

- It's common for your hands to swell while you are walking. If your hands do swell, remove your rings prior to your walk and don't wear anything tight around your wrists. Keep your hands slightly open and every so often stretch them out and make a fist. Holding them up or doing occasional arm circles can also help. Stay hydrated: drink water before, during, and after your walk.

CHITCHAT

The key to the success of this step is walking briskly. But *brisk* is a rather broad term, and I feel the need to explain what is meant by it. When I first embarked on my Simple Steps journey toward health, I walked at a brisk pace of three miles per hour (twenty minutes a mile). Depending on your fitness level, you may start at a higher or lower pace. As my fitness level increased, so did my walking pace. My brisk walking pace is now five miles per hour (twelve minutes a mile). On an exceptionally good day, I can walk at the brisk pace of six miles per hour (ten minutes a mile). Either of these speeds is equivalent to jogging, which you may find you prefer to do. But I like to walk fast, and I know that at my best pace I'm actually burning more calories. Simply put, when I walk briskly, I walk at a pace that causes my body to sweat. I know that sounds too simple, but listen to your body. If your body is sweating and your heart rate increases, you are walking at what we consider to be your brisk pace. Don't compare yourself with anyone—your fitness level is unique to your body, and your body's concept of *brisk* is just as unique.   —Beverly Zingarella

- Do not replace your daily walk with any other form of exercise. No matter what your exercise regime currently consists of (aerobics videos, exercise bike, etc.), enjoy the oxygen-enriching benefits gained from getting out into the fresh air to walk. So keep up your other activities and simply add twenty minutes of outdoor walking. It is important for this to become a new healthy habit.

The Key: Attaching This Step to Your Current Lifestyle

- Make this step the first thing you do every morning. Morning workouts are the ones you are least likely to skip because that time slot is least affected by errands or events that crop up as the day goes on.
- Keep your workout clothes next to your bed so you don't think twice about walking when you wake up.
- Get into the habit of parking farther away from your office or the shopping mall, or getting off your bus or train one stop early so you can walk to work.
- Instead of a coffee break, take a walking break.
- Find support. Partner up with a walking buddy or take your dog for a walk.
- Start a neighborhood walking club. Regular walking is a great way to find time to chat with friends or family.
- Get support from your family. After dinner, add more enjoyment to your daily walk by getting family members to join you. Walk with your spouse, or take a stroller walk with the baby. Not only will you digest your meal better, but walking is a fun and healthy family activity.

- Make your walk an adventure; seek out things you haven't noticed before. You will be amazed at how much you have never noticed in your own neighborhood.
- Mark a star on your calendar each day upon completing your walk. Seeing all of those stars will help keep you motivated.
- If you find your own unique way to attach this step to your personal lifestyle, please share your ideas with us on our Web site: www.SimpleStepsProgram.com.

Drawers, Cabinets, and Closets

Clean Out a Drawer, Cabinet, or Closet Every Week

Why Do We Need to Clean Out Drawers, Cabinets, and Closets?

- For most of us, having clean drawers, cabinets, and closets is stress reducing. Cleaning out even just the smallest drawer this week will serve as your first tangible household organizational step on the program, allowing you to clearly see the connection between clutter and stress, *de*-cluttering and *de*-stressing. Messy drawers, cabinets, and closets drain us of our energy.
- Organized drawers, cabinets, and closets will give us back precious time. We typically waste far too much time looking for misplaced items such as keys, scissors, eyeglasses, or even a favorite sweater.
- We'll be able to find what we need as these storage spaces become organized. We will probably be reunited with several items we had lost or forgotten about.
- If we're short on storage space in our home, we may find, after this de-cluttering step, we have more room for what we really use every day.

- Items in organized drawers and cabinets can be accessed easily. Nothing is more frustrating than reaching for the glass water pitcher and having to take out every mixing bowl and baking dish we own to get to it.
- Through our own research, we have come to the conclusion that for women, clutter and chaos in the home appear to be linked to eating as an emotional escape. There is a connection between organizing clutter and losing weight. So get busy!

How to Organize a Cluttered Drawer, Messy Cabinet, and Closet

- Where do you start? With the place that needs your attention most: the kitchen junk drawer or cluttered medicine cabinet, the laundry cabinet or your linen closet. It really doesn't matter; the bottom line is to just get started.
- Imagine your home completely uncluttered and orderly. Visualize your kitchen drawers that are only one layer deep with kitchen tools, so you don't have to dig for everything you need. Picture your bathroom cabinets stacked with neatly folded sets of fresh, matching bathroom towels, and so on.
- Now, a bit of strategic planning. Once you've chosen the drawer or cabinet to work on, decide exactly what this storage space is to be used for. Your answer is usually determined by location. For instance, a drawer near an entrance to your home may be used to hold keys and sunglasses; a drawer near a telephone should hold notepads, pens, and phone book; and baking needs should be organized in a cabinet near the oven.
- Set a timer. Give yourself a half hour to complete the task and it won't overwhelm you, no matter how cluttered that first drawer is. If you can't finish in a half hour, just continue the job for a

half hour tomorrow. Remember, you can take the whole week for one drawer if you have to. *No* job is too much for us if we break it into Simple Steps.

A DRAWER

- If you decide to tackle a cluttered drawer, you must take the drawer completely out and empty all the contents of the drawer onto the counter, the floor, a bed, or a table.
- When the drawer is completely empty, take this opportunity to wipe clean the inside with warm water. Use a little baking soda to remove anything sticky. You may even want to line the drawer with Con-Tact paper for a pretty perk and to make future cleaning jobs easier.
- When cleaning out the drawer that holds your forks, spoons, and knives, don't forget to take out the divider tray that holds them and wash it. You'll be amazed by how dirty it's gotten.
- Find two empty shoe boxes (or similar sized bins) and a brown paper shopping bag. Apply the Simple Steps golden rule of sorting: RECYCLE, RELOCATE, and DISCARD. The first shoe box is for recycling items that will go back into that drawer. The second shoe box is for relocating those items that need to find new homes elsewhere in your household. The brown paper bag is for discarding the stuff that belongs in the garbage. If you don't need it, if you do not know what it is, or if it's been broken for far too long, just get rid of it. (Which is the reason we suggest a brown bag—you can't see through it. Don't open up the bag to look inside once the task is completed. You might get tempted to rescue some of your unnecessary junk.)
- To organize the drawer, place shallow, small boxes inside to house loose items, such as pens, combs and brushes, or arts and crafts supplies.

- Test all pens contained in drawers and make sure they write. Sharpen all pencils.
- Put a dryer fabric softener sheet into the back of the drawer to produce a fresh scent, or try an old-fashioned sachet.
- After putting the drawer back into its tracks, remember to take five minutes and walk around your home, delivering the items from your relocate box to proper locations. After all, your son's plastic dinosaur toy really didn't need to be in your office desk drawer.

A CABINET

- If you choose to organize a messy cabinet this week, empty the entire contents onto a counter or a table.
- Don't forget to wipe clean the cabinet shelves. Now is the time to install shelving paper if you so choose.
- Decide how sections of the cabinet will be used. All items should be with like items—plasticware together, baking needs together, canned food together, and so on.
- Again, apply the Simple Steps golden rule of sorting: You need one place to put any items to be returned to that cabinet, another place for items to be moved to an alternate cabinet (remember to store items with like items), and a third place for items to be tossed into the garbage or given away.
- When restocking the cabinet, always place your frequently used items in the front and your moderately used items in the back.
- Relocate the items that go in other cabinets and discard your unneeded items.
- Expandable shelf organizers are great for creating extra storage in awkward spaces, such as under the kitchen sink.
- If you've chosen to organize your dish cabinet, remember that you need only one set of everyday dishes in your kitchen. Dis-

card any chipped or old pieces just collecting dust. Get rid of the old glasses and mugs you never use.

- Apply the one-year rule to all household clutter. Look at everything in the cabinet, from kitchen gadgets to old worn-out towels. If you haven't used it in the past year, toss it. If you can't bear to throw it away, pass it on to a friend, sell it at a yard sale, or donate it to charity.

- If you are finding it difficult to part with your frivolous things because of emotional reasons, simply pack them up into a box, seal it, date it six months from today (mark your calendar too) and place it out of sight in your attic, basement, or garage. When you reach the date in your calendar marked "the box in basement," retrieve the box and remove it from your home without looking inside it. You obviously can live without it. You proved to your emotional side that you really do not need what is in there anymore.

A CLOSET

- When emptying the contents of a closet, you might want to begin sorting as you are emptying it. Use our three-pile sorting system right on the floor in front of the closet: one pile for those things beautiful, useful, and loved; the second pile for those items to be put away elsewhere; and the third pile for items going to the trash or being given away.

- Make better use of two typically wasted closet spaces: the space over the clothing rod (sometimes adding an extra shelf up there makes good sense), and the space under the hanging clothes (shoe racks or storage bins with drawers offer a smart solution).

- Large storage bins in closets are helpful. Remember to label the contents.

- Many of us have a closet cluttered with wrapping paper. Organize your holiday or everyday wrap efficiently with a two-sided hanging gift wrap organizer that fits easily in even a small hall closet. The organizer takes up only about as much room as a suit jacket. Each side has pockets to hold rolls of gift wrap, ribbons, gift bags, etc.

· Linen closet: Try packing a complete sheet set into its matching pillowcase for quick access and a neater look.

CHITCHAT

It is important to develop efficient systems of organization for each drawer, cabinet, and closet so they will not get disorganized again and again. One method I find that works is to determine which items are used on a daily basis, which items are used on a somewhat frequent basis, and which items are hardly ever used at all. Do not crowd your precious kitchen space (typically the hub of a household) with items you do not need daily. Any household items that are hardly used at all can easily be contained in a labeled bin and stored in the basement, attic, or garage. I recently cleared out two of the kitchen drawers I realized I seldom open. They were filled with household batteries, camera film, and lightbulbs. Although these are necessary household items, I certainly do not use them on a daily basis in my kitchen. I realized I was wasting valuable kitchen space, so I found two small empty drawers in a back laundry room to house these items instead. —Lisa Lelas

The Key: Attaching This Step to Your Current Lifestyle

· Dedicate a time each week for drawer, cabinet, or closet cleanup. Mark it on your calendar to help you stick with it.
· So you're not tempted to retrieve a discarded item, plan your drawer-, cabinet-, or closet-cleaning time around garbage pickup days or visits to your selected charity.
· Put a reminder note on the refrigerator: "Have you cleaned a drawer today?"
· Make organizing your drawer, cabinet, or closet a part of your weekly cleaning routine. Every Friday, for instance, pull out a drawer and get to work. Eventually, after all of your household drawers and cabinets are completely in order (true nirvana), you can continue with simple maintenance checks. Remember that *keeping up* is easier than *catching up*. Even if it takes you all week to clean that first drawer, an organized system will spare you from having to spend that much time keeping it clean.

WEIGHT LOSS TIP

Try to schedule your de-clutter project during the time of day when you're typically the most hungry, and the most likely to snack. Keeping your focus away from food for just twenty minutes can remove you completely from a hunger cycle.

· Keep your drawers, cabinets, and closets organized on a daily basis by returning contents to their proper place after using them.

- For moms with kids at home, try having a two-minute tidy-up race. Set the kitchen timer for two minutes at the same time every day (at four p.m., or just before dinner, for example) and have everyone race to put away things (toys, craft supplies, etc.) in the drawer, cabinet, closet, or bin where they belong. You'll be amazed at how quickly you can get clutter put away, even with the help of very small hands.

> ## ORGANIZING TIP
>
> Gather everyone in your household together and explain the function of the household storage spaces. Ask them to commit to keeping these spaces clutter free. Getting your family involved in the organization of your home is very important in maintaining its order.

- Stop bringing unnecessary clutter into your home. If you are not a naturally organized person, the best way to manage your mess is simply to have less of it!
- If you find your own unique way to attach this step to your personal lifestyle, please share your ideas with us on our Web site: www.SimpleStepsProgram.com.

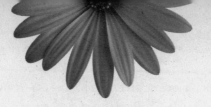

Money

Start Saving $2 a Day (or at Least 1 Percent of Your Weekly Salary After Taxes, Whichever Is Greater)

Why Do We Need to Save Money?

- Money is one of the biggest stress inducers. Gaining control of our finances is the first step to financial freedom.
- The National Center for Women and Retirement Research points out that 80–90 percent of all women will be solely responsible for their own finances at some point in their life.
- Women make less money (33 percent less) than men over their lifetime, according to the National Center of Women and Retirement. The average annual income for a female older than sixty-five is less than $7,000.
- According to the National Center for Women and Retirement Research, the average age for a woman to be widowed is fifty-five. Seventy-five percent of our elderly poor are women. Eighty percent of widows now living in poverty were not poor before their husbands died. To protect our own security, it is vital to start gaining control of our finances.
- We believe that every woman should have enough money within

her control to move out and rent a place of her own—even if she never wants to or never needs to!

How to Save Money

- An easy way to begin is to clean out an empty coffee can or juice bottle (with the top glued on) to use as your rainy-day bank. Watch how fast $2 a day can accumulate.
- You say you can't afford to save $2 a day? Try saving just 1 percent of your weekly salary. If you make $10,000 a year after taxes, 1 percent of your weekly salary equals $1.92 per day.
- When your rainy-day bank reaches $150, think about transferring the cash to a passbook savings plan at your local bank.
- Balance your checkbook, examine your credit card statements, and take stock of where your money is being spent. Review the last six months and make a list of the places your money usually goes. Figure out the average you spend in each category each month. Line up all the information, and you have your first budget. Can you afford your lifestyle? If not, cut what you can until your budget works. If you have any extra, figure out what you can save. Maybe it's more than $2 a day!
- If you are married and your husband does the household finances, sit down with him and learn what he does. Finding out where your money is going will help you to recognize where you can save.
- Use a debit card, not a credit card. With a debit card you can spend only up to the amount you have in the bank.
- Clean out your purse and wallet: Sort your money, organizing bills in a neat and proper order from large bills to small, not crumpled up throughout your purse. Financial advisor Suze Orman says she can tell who is wealthy or can become wealthy

just by the organizational condition of his or her wallet. She believes you must respect money to have money enter and stay in your life.

- Save any change you find after cleaning out your drawer or cabinet this week.
- Say no to one impulse purchase every day. Making small adjustments can add to your savings.
- Learn the difference between wanting and needing. We need food, not a gourmet meal.
- Shop with a list and stick to it. Never go grocery shopping while you are hungry.
- Use coupons.
- Trade baby-sitting services with friends and neighbors.
- Brew your own pot of coffee. Instead of buying a cup of java at the local café, put away that cash. Just 97 cents a day, the average cost of a cup of coffee, adds up to over $29 a month, points out personal finance expert Michelle Hoesley.
- If you eat dinner out once a week, make it once a month.
- Try the no-spend cold turkey challenge: For one week, or even a three-day period, try not to spend one penny. Every time you reach to buy a magazine or a cup of coffee or a new outfit—or consider driving through a car wash—write down the amount you would have spent. You will be amazed at how high the figure is at the end of the week.
- Involve the whole family. Ask your husband and kids to contribute spare change. Think of a reward, such as a family dinner at the kids' favorite restaurant, when the agreed-upon goal is reached.

CHATTER TIME

Barbara, a recent Simple Steps participant, shared a true story of how small savings made a dramatic difference in her family's life. Barbara and her husband were trying desperately to save money for their first home. After years of saving, the couple was told by the bank they needed an additional $30,000 for their down payment. They had no other option but to ask Barbara's parents to co-sign a loan. Barbara was shocked when her mom called her into the bedroom and revealed a secret savings box in her closet containing over $120,000. "This is forty-five years' worth of spare change," her mother boasted to her. "Even your father has no idea!"

The Key: Attaching This Step to Your Current Lifestyle

- Every day upon returning home from work, get into the habit of throwing your loose pocket change into your rainy-day bank.
- Every evening after dinner, prepare a bagged school lunch for your child and save approximately $300 annually. Save even more by preparing a bagged lunch for yourself to bring to work.
- At the end of each week, stop and count how much rainy-day money you've saved. And do it again at the end of every month. You'll be delighted.
- Each week put aside the money you saved from using coupons at the grocery store. Every few weeks purchase a U.S. savings bond with the money you have accumulated.
- Make a plan of how you'll spend your rainy-day money at the

end of the year. Do you want to invest it? Go on a shopping spree? It's up to you. But knowing what you're saving for will help you make this step a habit.

- If you find your own unique way to attach this step to your personal lifestyle, please share your ideas with us on our Web site: www.SimpleStepsProgram.com.

Sharing

Overcoming Tragedy with Creative
Refocusing and Newfound Support:
A Story of Hope

Michele sat quietly observing the circle of twelve seemingly confident women. She was one of the first members of the Simple Steps
program, a new lifestyle makeover workshop started in her New
England community. Michele listened as the three bubbly codirec-
tors walked the women through the basic guidelines of the program
with the promise to help them refocus, reenergize, and live a
healthier, more positive life.

A more positive life? Michele thought sadly. Maybe for the rest
of them, but certainly not for me. They would never understand
what I have been through.

Michele admits she joined Simple Steps only after some coaxing
by a good friend. "Go ahead; it will be good for you," she had been
told. "You need to get out and start living again." Michele knew she
had put on a few pounds and thought a healthy-lifestyle check
might be good for her, but as far as refocusing and recharging went,
she just couldn't see that happening anytime soon. How could she
ever open up to this group of strangers? she wondered. They
couldn't possibly understand. It was all too painful.

Michele remembered that dreadful day, the day her husband,
Steve, called her from a business trip, crying. "Something is

wrong," he said. "I don't feel well. I'm coming home." That phone call marked the beginning of the tragedy that sent Michele's life into a tailspin.

Michele and Steve, both in their late thirties, had been happily married for twelve years. They were a beautiful couple, both Italian with rich, dark skin and hair. He was athletic and handsome, a successful salesman of audio equipment in New York. Michele was a friendly, whimsical woman, with a passion for interior decorating and arts and crafts. The only thing missing in their lives was a child. After years of trying, when Michele still couldn't get pregnant, she started taking fertility drugs. When that didn't work, Michele and Steve tried in vitro fertilization. The couple celebrated when doctors told them their baby was on the way.

Two months after their daughter, Alex, was born, Steve started experiencing frightening symptoms. His speech was slurred and his arm muscles twitched. Doctors assured him nothing was wrong, and when Steve began seeing a psychologist, convinced he must be creating his own physical problems, the psychologist, too, told him he was fine. Still, the symptoms got worse. He started tripping and falling while walking. Finally, because of Steve's persistence, doctors came up with a diagnosis: Steve had Lou Gehrig's disease, or ALS, a fatal disease with no known treatment or cure. The disease was attacking the nerve cells in his brain and spinal cord. Doctors weren't sure how long he would live. They gave him anywhere from two weeks to ten years.

Michele reeled with fear and anxiety, knowing her husband was dying. Steve tried to work, but the disease progressed rapidly. It wasn't long before he was paralyzed, unable to walk or speak. He could barely use his hands and had to be fed through a feeding tube. Michele watched him deteriorate and exhausted herself caring for him. "He was my number one," she told friends. "Even the baby came second. I had no energy left for me." She tried to ease her husband's suffering, with no time to coddle the baby she had waited so long for.

When Michele fell into bed every night, she worried about how much longer they could afford their house. Though Steve had a successful career, they had never invested in health insurance. They hadn't thought they would need it so soon; after all, Michele and Steve were both still in their thirties. They had spent so much money trying to get pregnant, and with Michele now staying home to care for her family, there was no income. They relied on friends and relatives pitching in to put food on the table. Their community held an art auction to help pay her husband's medical bills.

More than two years passed. Steve communicated to Michele with a special computer, and one day he spelled out this message for Michele: "It's over." He died in her arms an hour later. Alex, their baby girl, was only three years old.

For a year and a half following Steve's death, all Michele could do was eat, sleep, and undergo counseling; it was all she could manage. She fell into a deep depression. She didn't understand why she would be blessed with a baby, only to lose her husband. Michele fell apart both psychologically and physically. She knew she had been gaining weight, but didn't care. She couldn't think about doing anything for herself, not even socializing.

Eventually, a friend who had been there for her throughout Steve's illness told her about Simple Steps. Michele realized that she had come to a point of wanting to feel better. She knew she had to do something, if not for herself, then for her daughter.

When she first joined the focus group, she had doubts, but Michele promised herself she would finish the program; she had made the commitment. By the end of the first week's session, she realized that the other twelve women also had their own stories. Some were there to lose a lot of weight; a few just needed to shed those last stubborn 15 pounds. Others needed to reorganize, find personal time, de-stress and de-clutter. A few, like Michele, had endured painful hardships. She was touched by one woman's delight at the first tufts of hair growing back on her head; she was a breast cancer survivor. Michele related to her and shared her own story with the group.

It was a triumph for Michele just to be there with other people. Little by little, things began to change. She felt better when she came to the meetings and listened to the other women. She did the Simple Steps halfheartedly at first, but soon she welcomed them as a part of her daily routine. She drank her water from a pretty long-stem wineglass. She lit a candle at dinner and by her bath.

When she'd been given her first small de-clutter assignment, Michele reported back to the group that she had cleaned out an amazing sixteen drawers and cabinets in her home. Her new circle of friends applauded with encouragement. The de-clutter project focused her energy on something she felt she could have some control over, and it made her feel better about herself. She realized in the process that she had been neglecting herself for years. Simple Steps was teaching her how to do nice things for herself. She started looking forward to seeing the other women in her group, to sharing all of their accomplishments of the week.

Michele knew she had crossed a major threshold when she made a treasure map as a part of the Simple Steps program. She was instructed to cut out pictures or images from magazines that represented her goals. She was drawn to a picture of a beautiful woman being kissed on the cheek by a man. It had been almost two years since her husband's death. She had not entertained the thought of remarrying or even dating, but she couldn't stop looking at the picture. She cut it out of the magazine, and though feeling slightly embarrassed and even a bit guilty, she held it up at the meeting, took a deep breath, and surprised herself as she said these words: "I want to find love again." Tears rolled down her cheeks. A few of the

women started to cry out of happiness for her, while others applauded loudly. Michele remembers feeling so relieved; everyone
was thrilled for her. She started thinking about making plans for
her life. She didn't want to be alone forever.

Michele knew at that moment that she was on her way to starting
to live again. With the help of the Simple Steps program, she had finally come to understand that there was a purpose for her. As
Michele sums it up, "I came to understand Steve was a significant
chapter in my life. I can't ever forget that. I'm stronger and more
assertive now." She's now grateful that a part of Steve still survives
in their daughter.

Michele believes it was the support of the twelve women in her
Simple Steps group that truly helped lift her out of some of her
toughest, darkest days. She realized that there were people out
there who cared about her and were there to listen to and encourage
her. "I know now I have to take care of myself and that I'm ready for
the next chapter in my life."

Congratulations!

You've now mastered the following Simple Steps. Read them aloud as a positive affirmation. Make them a habit and keep them up as part of your new lifestyle.

I am drinking eight cups of water daily

I am walking twenty minutes a day

I am clearing out one drawer/cabinet/closet space every week

I am saving $2 a day (or 1 percent of my weekly salary)

The Daisy

A symmetrical beauty.
An early spring bloomer,
she is reliable and familiar,
abundant and inviting.

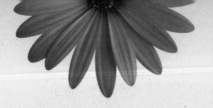

Food Journaling

Write Down What You Eat and How It Makes You Feel

Why Should We Keep a Food Journal?

- Writing down our food intake helps us analyze our diet to be sure we are eating healthfully. Keeping a food diary will help us realistically gauge our calorie consumption. A recent study published in *The New England Journal of Medicine* found that when people wrote down what they ate, they realized they had been underestimating their consumption by an average of 1,053 calories a day.
- Writing may be just what we need to lose extra pounds, says eDiets.com psychologist Dr. Susan Mendelsohn. Dr. Mendelsohn sees writing as an alternative to eating when we need to keep your hands busy. Journaling will also help us release pent-up feelings rather than stuffing them down with food. Venting through journaling helps cravings pass more constructively.
- Two of the most powerful tools around are the pen and paper, states Jeffrey Wilbert, Ph.D., author of *Fattitudes: Beat Self-Defeat and Win Your War with Weight*. According to Wilbert, research studies have shown that those most likely to lose weight and keep it off use a technique called self-monitoring. Self-

monitoring is keeping track of you—tuning in to your thoughts, feelings, goals, and strategies. You chart your own progress and reward yourself for successes. Wilbert suggests that monitoring include what you eat as well as why you eat. Identifying issues and feelings that trigger overeating is important.

- Keeping a food journal allows us to control the food rather than letting the food control us.

- If you *love* food, you could have an unhealthy emotional attachment, according to John H. Sklare, psychologist on eDiets.com. Remember, food is just nourishment.

- Food journaling can also help you pinpoint why you are suffering from various ailments. For example, if you have frequent headaches, tracking your food intake might provide answers as to why. Headaches can be the result of eating foods containing nitrates, caffeine, MSG, or artificial sweeteners.

- Food journaling makes meal planning easier. You will recognize your patterns of eating and be able to plan balanced meals with healthy snacks in between.

- We have found that keeping a journal has helped us learn to read labels and comprehend the caloric values of different foods.

- You may soon find that when you have to record in your journal a snack, a dessert, that café mocha, that second can of soda, or an extra helping, it doesn't seem worth eating after all.

How to Keep a Food Journal

- Take our challenge! Write down every single thing you put into your mouth: all the quick bites while you're cooking, the drinks, the leftovers on your children's plates, etc. With each entry, record your mood. You will be amazed to learn exactly what and how much you are eating, as well as how many times you eat for reasons other than hunger.

• Before eating anything, ask yourself, "Am I really hungry?" and "Do I really need this, and if so, why?" Answer these questions in your journal. If you crave a fattening food, ask yourself if you are hungry enough to eat instead a bowl of fresh carrots, celery, or another healthy food. If the thought of eating healthy food is not appealing to you, perhaps you are not really hungry.

• Be sure to write down what you eat right after you eat it. Don't trick yourself into saying that you will write everything down at the day's end. If you don't write it down immediately, you might forget.

• You may want to use a food scale or measuring cup until you learn appropriate serving sizes (see pages 15–16).

• To lose weight, you have to take in less food energy (calories) than you expend. You might want to use your food journal to keep track of how many calories you burn in your daily activities.

• Once you are aware of your particular eating patterns, plan a snack a short time before you are most at risk of bingeing.

• Identifying your mood patterns will help you deal with what is behind your emotional eating. Find a new way to cope with distress—perhaps walking, bicycle riding, or reading. Write down your feelings rather than stuffing them down with food.

The Key: Attaching This Step to Your Current Lifestyle

• Make it a point every morning to begin your day by dating the top of a new page in your food journal.

• Keep your journal with you all day. You probably will want to use a small notebook that can fit in your purse or pocket, or you can also put your journal in your calendar, daily planner, or Palm-Pilot. The idea is to make it portable enough to carry with you throughout the day.

· Keep your journal handy at each meal. The keys to keeping any sort of journal are accessibility and being totally open and honest. Write down everything you eat and your feelings. It might be intimidating at first, but you will soon see results from journaling.

· If you find your own unique way to attach this step to your personal lifestyle, please share your ideas with us on our Web site: www.SimpleStepsProgram.com.

Isometrics

Squeeze Some Isometrics Into Every Day

Why Should We Do Isometrics?

- Isometrics are a fun, easy, and inexpensive exercise program.
- These simple workouts can be done just about anywhere, anytime.
- No exercise equipment is needed to do isometrics.
- In just minutes a day, isometrics can help shape and tone our muscles.
- Isometrics isolate and work a specific problem area. Isometrics can thin our thighs, flatten our tummy, firm our buttocks, and tone our arms.
- Kegel exercises are considered a form of isometrics. These exercises are especially important for women who have given birth and want to tone their pelvic muscles, have more control of their bladder, and increase sexual pleasure. "Kegel exercises can strengthen the pelvic floor muscles and reduce your chances of a leak," says Dr. Deborah Erickson, M.D., a urologist and assistant professor of surgery at Pennsylvania State University, College of Medicine. These exercises are good for all women as we age.

How to Do Isometrics

- As with any other exercise program, consult your physician before starting up a new physical exercise routine. Isometrics tend to elevate blood pressure levels. People with hypertension, heart disease, or other medical problems may be warned not to practice isometrics.
- Isometrics are exercises without movement in which muscles are contracted and strengthened through resistance. For example, simply contract the muscles of your abdomen for ten seconds, tensing up as if someone were about to deliver a punch to that area. (You can practice now while you are reading this. If you are seated, press your back against the chair. After ten seconds, relax the muscles for a few seconds, and then repeat the pattern of contracting and relaxing five times. Work up to a set of six, ten times per day. The secret is to concentrate on isolating one muscle group at a time.
- Don't forget to breathe while you're doing isometrics. Breathe in when you tighten your muscles and exhale when you relax.
- To do Kegel exercises, for ten seconds contract your interior pelvic floor muscles as if you were holding in a full bladder, then relax. Do a set of ten, three times per day.
- To help tone your upper arms and chest, hold your hands together like you would if you were praying, keeping your hands right in front of your chest with your thumbs resting against your sternum. Press your hands together using all of your arm and chest muscles. Hold for a slow count of five, release, and repeat five times.
- Another great chest toner: Stand in a doorway with your hands at shoulder height and your palms out. Press your palms against the door frame. Hold for a slow count of five, release, and repeat five times. To work different muscles, repeat while drop-

ping your hands to your sides and pressing the backs of your hands against the door frame.

- For your buttocks and thighs, clench these muscles, hold for a slow count of five, release, and then repeat five times.
- Use isometrics to help firm up your chin area. Lift your chin slightly, resting your finger on the hollow of your neck, close your mouth, and gently apply pressure with your tongue to the roof of your mouth. Feel the muscle tighten and contract with your finger.

The Key: Attaching This Step to Your Current Lifestyle

- Use your commuting time to and from work to practice isometrics. We have our Simple Steps group participants hold in their abs or butt muscles every time they're in their car and stop at a red light. Hold the contracted muscles until the light changes to green.
- Every time you fill up your gas tank, do Kegel exercises until you hear the click of the gas pump telling you your tank is full.

CHITCHAT

I remember that when we first started the program, I decided to squeeze at red lights. I not only squeezed my abs, but I squeezed my arms, legs, buttocks, and anything else that needed to be squeezed, holding this position until the light turned green. One day, while sitting at a light in my "squeeze" position, I happened to notice the people in the car next to me were looking at me rather strangely—I hadn't realized that when I squeezed, I also made funny faces!

—Linda McClintock

- Each day target a different muscle group. For instance: Mondays are for abs, Tuesdays for buttocks, Wednesdays for thighs, Thursdays for upper arms, and Fridays for Kegels.
- While your coffee is brewing, do three sets of ten repetitions of isometrics. Feel free to rest for thirty seconds to one minute in between sets, if needed.

MORE CHITCHAT

In our Simple Steps group sessions, we've found that handing out stickers that say SQUEEZE works well to remind group members to do their daily isometrics. Many of them place the sticker on the steering wheel of their car as a reminder to do isometrics while they're on the road. Others opt for placing the sticker on their television remote control. You can use a simple label gun to create your own reminder sticker, or even post a plain paper note in various places.

—Beverly, Linda, and Lisa

- TV-time isometrics: Do isometrics during the first ad of every commercial break while watching television shows.
- Your day is filled with little moments during which you can practice isometrics: while brushing your teeth, waiting for the microwave to finish, talking on the phone, waiting for your bus or train, sitting at your desk, or waiting in a bank line. See how many moments you can find in your day.
- If you find your own unique way to attach this step to your personal lifestyle, please share your ideas with us on our Web site: www.SimpleStepsProgram.com.

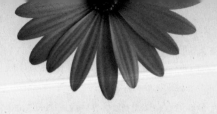

Laundry

Set Up an Efficient Laundry System

Why Should We Set Up a Laundry System?

- Most of the women in our groups report that laundry is a major clutter problem in households, adding stress to their lives. Clean, folded, and stored clothing is stress relieving.
- By setting up a regular laundry schedule, we spend less time doing laundry. It doesn't have to be a constant chore.
- By keeping up with laundry, we have all of our clothes where they are intended to be (not in the clothes hamper). We become aware of which items need to be repaired, which have stains to treat, or which need to be replaced because they no longer fit, no longer look good, or are simply worn-out.
- We can keep many stains from permanently setting by doing regular wash loads. Soiled spots can stain clothes left in hampers too long.

How to Set Up a Laundry System That Works

- No matter how much laundry you have, you can find a laundry system that works with your routine.
- Determine the laundry needs of your household. Do you have a large family with small kids? A family with teens who can do their own laundry? Is it just you and your spouse? Do you live alone? This will help you choose which laundry system is right for you.
- Generally, if you wash less than five loads of laundry per week, a one-day-a-week system should work for you. If you wash five loads or more per week, you might want to consider doing laundry for a short time each day.
- To implement a weekly wash system, you should establish one day of the week as your laundry day. On laundry day, all laundry must be washed, dried, folded, ironed (if needed), and put away. Block out sufficient time on that day to handle your loads.
- Remember, five loads take about five hours start to finish, but you don't have to sit and watch it spin in your machine. Plan a half hour at the start for sorting, and another at the end for folding and storing. During the remaining four hours, just pop in to change loads.
- If you do a lot of laundry and can't seem to keep the laundry baskets from overflowing, consider trying a daily system, for more manageable loads. To make this work, you must adhere to a strict morning or evening laundry routine (selecting an hour for one complete laundry cycle, wash to dry), or you will find yourself doing laundry throughout the day, defeating the purpose of an efficient system.
- Have ample clothes hampers. Picking clothes up off the floor shouldn't be the start of your laundry chores. One hamper for

CHITCHAT

Since establishing a daily laundry system in my house, I feel like I am never doing laundry anymore! My laundry chores have now become a part of my normal weekday routine. The loads are smaller and more manageable. Every evening before going to bed, I sort the contents of the clothes hampers and throw a load into the washer. Good night. Then, when I wake up to get ready for my morning walk, I take the load out of the washer and throw it into the dryer or hang it to drip-dry. By the time I eat my breakfast, I have already folded and put away the clothes that were sitting in the hampers just last night! Occasionally I will have a second daily wash (delicates, all whites, etc.) that I also try to fit in before breakfast, but for the most part, the rest of my day begins laundry free! —Lisa Lelas

each bedroom and bathroom is suggested. Assign a laundry basket to each family member, and consider purchasing divided clothes hampers to encourage family members to separate their dirty clothes by color. Laundry is quicker and easier when clothes are already separated.

· For families with children, the key to reducing your laundry time is having clothes that can be washed together without fear of colors running and do not need to be ironed.

· Save time by checking labels when you buy clothes. Does the item need to be dry-cleaned, ironed, or hand washed? If so, consider how much more time or money will go into laundering that item.

· Create a clothing repair center for all clothing items that need a button, alteration, or mending. If possible, do all of your mending in one sitting, or bring your mending to a tailor to save time.

· Have a separate basket or drawstring bag for your dry cleaning items. Visit the dry cleaner on the same day of each week to simplify your routine. Don't forget to return those wire hangers!

· Be sure to keep a full stock of laundry supplies: detergent, spot remover, bleach, fabric softener, a mending kit, laundry baskets, extra hangers, and a drying rack. Arrange your laundry products from left to right in the order that you use them.

· Keep a small toothbrush and cheap bottle of shampoo in your laundry room for scrubbing noticeable stains. It's a lot cheaper than buying expensive stain remover sticks and gels.

· Keep the products you need near the washer so you have them at your fingertips. If you don't have the room, try using a rolling caddy that slides in between your washer and dryer.

· Place a pretty decorative dish by the washer/dryer to hold items you find in pants pockets, such as coins or loose buttons.

· Your laundry room should be bright and easy to clean. Try adding a few comfort items such as a soft rug to stand on, a CD player, or even some framed photographs.

CHATTER TIME

Iris, a native of England and longtime Simple Steps follower, insists that line drying is simply the best way to get the freshest, cleanest-smelling clothes. She tells us that she searches her home for any clothes to wash on a good line-drying day, even if it's not her typical laundry day. "I hate to waste a windy day!" she admits.

- Recent research indicates that all bed linens should be laundered every week to eliminate dust mites, which commonly cause allergic reactions. Linens should be not only tended to weekly but washed in a hot temperature and dried on high, for a double dose of heat (the only way proven to get rid of the dust mite eggs that might otherwise be hidden in the fibers). If you prefer the fresh smell of line-dried linens, wash and dry them first, then hang them outside.

- For the most part, you should always wash clothes in warm or hot water. Detergents work best in water that is warmer than 65 degrees. Turn dark items inside out to help prevent fading.

- Don't load your washer too full. Clothes get cleaner with more water circulating between them.

- Don't overload your dryer. Your clothes will get wrinkled and take longer to dry.

- For quicker and more efficient drying cycles, keep the lint filter cleaned out. Clean it out after every load that is dried. For multiple loads of laundry, drying one load right after the other conserves the heat remaining in the dryer.

- Eliminate the ironing basket. If your dryer does not buzz when the load is completed, set a small kitchen timer to let you know when the load should be done, and remove clothes from the dryer and hang them up as soon as possible to avoid wrinkles. For clothes you must iron, do it right away and then put them away.

- Set up a regular folding zone where you will feel comfortable and efficient, whether it be a kitchen table, a bed, a counter, or even the top of the washer/dryer. Make sure you are comfortable and not straining your back, especially if you have multiple loads to fold.

- Get into the habit of bringing empty hangers back into the laundry room for convenience.

- Get your family to take part in your new efficient laundry system. Have your children take their own dirty clothes to the laundry room or put them in a laundry bag or clothes hamper. Your children can also help fold some of the small towels, or at least help match socks, while you fold the rest of the clothes. Teamwork is a good lesson here.

The Key: Attaching This Step to Your Current Lifestyle

- Try incorporating small segments of your laundry duties in your regular routine, for example, by folding and putting away clothes right after you clear the breakfast dishes.
- Try folding your clothes after each load instead of at the end of the laundry day, or you might feel overwhelmed by a mountain of clothes to fold if you wash more than five loads.
- Throw a load of wash in every evening after brushing your teeth and, like Lisa, dry them first thing in the morning.
- If you find your own unique way to attach this step to your personal lifestyle, please share your ideas with us on our Web site: www.SimpleStepsProgram.com.

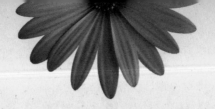

Daily Planning

SIMPLE STEP 8

Plan a To-Do List for Every Day

Why Should We Follow a To-Do List?

- We can conquer any task if we do it in small Simple Steps. A to-do list reminds us of that.
- We feel better having a direction, a way of organizing our responsibilities into achievable daily tasks. Daily planning is stress relieving.
- We use our time more efficiently when we work with a list that helps us prioritize activities, and we don't waste any time wondering, what else did I have to do?
- We learn how we're really spending our time when we review our to-do lists.
- When we plan ahead, manage our time more effectively, and follow to-do lists, we can begin to feel in control of our days, and of our lives. We can start seeing the bigger picture, that what we do today might help us accomplish a goal tomorrow.
- As author Ab Jackson says in her audiobook, *How to Organize Your Life and Get Rid of Clutter*, "The thirty smartest minutes of anyone's day is their planning time."

How to Start and Stick to a Daily To-Do List

GETTING STARTED

- If you are not sure where your time goes during the day, sketch out a twenty-four-hour pie chart and have each slice represent one hour of your day. Fill in "slices" according to where you currently spend your time each day. You may find the pie slices for family time are a lot fewer than those for your office time, or that TV time is more than you thought and your fitness time is barely noticeable. See where you can make adjustments to find more balance in your life. You might be surprised at how your time is spent.

- Some of us prefer to keep just one list. If you separate your office priority list from your personal priority list, in a pinch for time, the personal list gets disregarded.

- Others of us prefer to keep several to-do lists: for work, home, our kids, shopping, etc. If this is more comfortable for you, just be sure not to neglect any one list. (You might also want to use a personal digital assistant, like a PalmPilot, which usually allows you to separate or combine several different lists.)

- Your daily list can be written on loose pages, in a special to-do notebook or calendar, in a professional-style daily planner, or in a personal digital assistant.

- If you use a scrap sheet of paper or a simple notebook for your lists, make sure you carry it with you throughout the day and keep it out where you can see it. Folding the paper and simply throwing it into your purse is obviously not the best way to be reminded of your tasks.

- Always use the same kind of paper and layout on the page for all your to-do lists, so they will become a standard organizational tool you recognize and use. You don't want to take time to reinvent the format every morning.

COMPOSING YOUR DAILY LIST

- We recommend ordering your list according to the priority of the tasks. The tasks that need to be done first should be at the top.
- Don't let your list get too long. It will overwhelm you. You might want to keep a master list—all your jobs, chores, and concerns— and a separate shorter list of what you want to get done *today*. And don't put more on today's list than you can comfortably manage. Remember, there's always tomorrow!
- You can make the most of your daily list by writing in helpful details, such as your dentist's phone number next to the appointment time, or simple reminders, such as "Don't forget to pack the birthday gift."
- For errands and appointments, multitask. Try to batch similar tasks together to help you save time. For instance, when you have a doctor's appointment scheduled, stop at the dry cleaner if it's on the way to the doctor's office. Or if you're at home waiting for furniture to be delivered, schedule the plumber to come fix that leaky faucet.
- Sometimes it is helpful to include a projected date for completion of a particular task if it will run into several days or weeks. For instance: "Finish painting the family room by Saturday," or "Finish the book before the movie comes out on Thanksgiving Day."
- Once a week or once a month, pick a day to schedule an important appointment and mark it on your calendar: a mammogram, a teeth cleaning, a consultation with your accountant, etc. It doesn't matter if the appointment is months from now; you

will still feel less burdened by finally having that appointment scheduled.

- Before deciding what your basic goals are for the day, take a moment to reflect upon your true desires (what we call the bigger picture). Where do you see yourself by week's end? By year's end? Having a clear picture of what you want for yourself and developing a strategy for attaining that will help you determine what might be most important on your to-do list.

- Make your "self time" a priority on your to-do list by including your daily walk, a lunch with a friend, or an aerobics class at the gym.

COMPLETING YOUR TO-DO-LIST TASKS

- Stay focused. Try to limit interruptions. Make a conscious choice to stick with a particular task until the job is done. Have a coworker take your calls at the office or turn off the phone ringer in your home.

- If you do not complete a task on a particular day, make sure you log it in for the next day.

- If you consistently roll over uncompleted tasks to the following day, cut your to-do list in half so it will be more feasible to accomplish everything.

- Remember, you don't personally have to perform every task on your list. Ask family and coworkers for help.

- At the end of this first week, review your list. Note if and when you fell behind schedule and which days ran smoothly enough for you to check off all tasks as completed. Then decide how many activities, errands, appointments, and meetings you realistically are able to manage on a daily basis. You'll get more efficient at planning next week's lists.

The Key: Attaching This Step to Your Current Lifestyle

- Make your daily planning time a regular part of your day. For example, keep your daily planner on your nightstand each evening and map out the next day before going to sleep. Or wake up fifteen minutes earlier in the morning to make your list.
- At the breakfast table, recruit family members to help you complete various household tasks.
- Learn to say no. Politely decline requests for your time if they interfere with family time, or an important work project.
- Eat before or after the noontime lunch hour, so you can tackle some items on your list when your office is quiet.
- Limit your television watching. Finish one of your tasks instead of watching another rerun.
- Put an *X* on your calendar to mark your free time one day a month, or even one day every week. Don't schedule anything on those days marked with an *X*.
- If you find your own unique way to attach this step to your personal lifestyle, please share your ideas with us on our Web site: www.SimpleStepsProgram.com.

CHATTER TIME

Donna, a Simple Steps group participant, has finally found the balance she was seeking through careful weekly planning—or, actually, *not* planning. For more than a year now, she has gotten into the habit of taking a day off . . . from everything! On her kitchen calendar, she places an *X* on every Monday throughout the year. She plans nothing on Mondays: no haircuts, no grocery shopping, no doctor's appointments, and no after-school activities for the kids. She and her children enjoy Family Mondays, a free day to do whatever they feel like doing!

Sharing

By losing 54 Pounds and Quitting Smoking
on the Simple Steps Program, Jennifer
Learned to Love Herself Again

Thirty-nine-year-old Jennifer looked at her reflection in the mirror one day and didn't recognize the woman she saw. She remembered a time when she thought of herself as pretty and petite, accomplished and happy with herself. The person who stared back at her now from the mirror was 65 pounds overweight and wearing stretch pants. She wore stretch pants every day. It was the only thing left in her closet that still fit her.

It wasn't just the extra pounds that disturbed her. After eight years without a cigarette, Jennifer had started smoking again. She yelled at the kids, fought with her husband, and then brought a bowl of ice cream to bed every night to console herself.

And now, on the brink of her fortieth birthday, as she stared at the mirror, she felt afraid and alone. Jennifer knew in her heart that the woman she was looking at did not reflect who she really was inside. This was not her true self. Somewhere along the way she'd lost the Jennifer she loved, and another woman stood in her place. She knew she needed help but did not know where to turn.

A few weeks later, Jennifer noticed an article in her local newspaper that reached out and grabbed her. Three women in her hometown were starting a lifestyle makeover group. Their forty-step, ten-week program was called Simple Steps. She liked what she read. These three moms had created a new approach to weight loss, healthy living, de-cluttering, and reducing stress.

Jennifer responded and was one of the twenty-three women selected for a trial focus group. Together, the group members committed to meeting once a week and incorporating the Simple Steps into their daily lives, adding four steps every week.

Well, Simple Step by Simple Step, Jennifer was one of many in that group who experienced a dramatic transformation. She dropped 30 pounds in the first ten-week session and gave up smoking. She quickly signed up for another ten-week round and continued to lose the pounds. In just twenty weeks, she had lost 54 pounds and ten dress sizes.

"The weight started coming off because I wasn't focusing on food anymore," remembers Jennifer. "I was putting my energy into other things. I started walking. I started organizing my house. I was slowly de-stressing myself. As I went through the program, I realized that I really had been last on my priority list. I've learned that I am important. I've got my self-esteem and confidence back."

Jennifer's twelve-year-old daughter, Emily, beams proudly now, saying that her mom has shown her you have to take care of yourself to be happy.

In May of 2001, Jennifer was one of several Simple Steps participants selected to appear on *The Oprah Winfrey Show*. As a surprise to the other participants and the founding directors, the show gave her a head-to-toe makeover, from a new sassy hairstyle all the way down to new shoes. Tears of joy ran down the faces of her friends as Oprah showed photos of the old Jennifer and then welcomed the new and improved version on stage! All this, just ten days prior to her fortieth birthday.

"I couldn't have asked for a better birthday present." Jennifer smiles. "We really do get better with age. I know I did."

Today, Jennifer has still kept her weight off and remains a non-smoker. She continues walking daily and she takes Pilates exercise classes a few times per week. Her newfound energy enables her to keep up with her passions: sailing with her husband and daughters, gardening, cooking, and enjoying the beach when the weather is nice.

Congratulations!

You've now mastered the following Simple Steps. Read them aloud as a positive affirmation. Make them a habit and keep them up as part of your new lifestyle.

I am drinking eight cups of water daily

I am walking twenty minutes a day

I am clearing out one drawer/cabinet/closet space weekly

I am saving $2 a day (or 1 percent of my weekly salary)

I am keeping a daily food journal

I am squeezing in some isometrics every day

I am maintaining an efficient laundry system

I am following a daily to-do list

The Rose

Confident. Beautiful and radiant.
The classic symbol of pure beauty.

Vitamins

Take a Multivitamin Every Day

Why Should We Take a Multivitamin?

- A multivitamin is a simple way to give our body what it needs to function at its best and keep healthy.
- Eighty-eight percent of Americans exhibit poor eating habits as defined by *Dietary Guidelines for Americans*, developed by the U.S. Department of Agriculture (USDA), according to Michael Sacher, D.O., FACP, FACC. Even if we think we're eating foods rich in vitamins, overcooked and processed foods may have depleted levels of these essential vitamins and minerals.
- Getting the right amount of nutrients can help us defend against everything from heart disease to cancer.
- Calcium is a very important mineral for women. The calcium and vitamin D found in multivitamins are important for fighting osteoporosis.
- Caffeine depletes our body's stored calcium supply. Cutting down on the java and flushing out caffeine with water helps, but additional calcium from a multivitamin can do even more to help restore our needed calcium levels.
- Many multivitamins contain iron, an important mineral for

women, who are often anemic. Check with your doctor to find
out if an iron supplement is right for you.

· Multivitamins also contain antioxidants, such as vitamin C, vitamin E, and beta-carotene, which protect us from the forma-
tion of free radicals (by-products generated by our body that
can damage our cells).

· Selenium, another antioxidant found in a multivitamin, also
plays a role in activating the thyroid hormone, which regulates
the rate of our metabolism.

· Take a look at the Vitamin Guide to see the full range of benefits
we can enjoy from healthy amounts of vitamins and minerals.

VITAMIN GUIDE

NUTRIENT	BENEFIT	DAILY DOSAGE	SOURCES
Vitamin A	Maintains eyes, skin, teeth, and bones	800 mcg	Carrots, pumpkins, spinach, sweet potatoes, mangoes
Vitamin D	Teeth, bones; helps maintain calcium levels in blood	5–10 mcg	Salmon, oysters, milk, eggs, butter, yogurt, cheese
Vitamin E	Healthy tissue; protects red blood cells; antioxidant	8 mg	Vegetable oils, nuts, wheat germ, seeds, mangoes, olives

Vitamin K	Blood clotting; formation of bone	65 mcg	Brussels sprouts, kale, lettuce, spinach, broccoli
Vitamin C	Gums, bones; antioxidant to help fight infections; enhances absorption of iron	60 mg	Citrus fruit, papayas, kiwi, strawberries, red peppers, potatoes, tomatoes, broccoli
Folate	Heart; prevents birth defects	180 mcg	Fortified rice, pasta, bread, cereal; poultry; lentils, beans; leafy green vegetables
Thiamin (B1)	Muscle tone; digestion; helps cells convert carbohydrates into energy	1.1 mg	Yeast, pork, nuts, fish, soy, peas, beans, oatmeal, whole grains
Riboflavin (B2)	Skin; eyes; aids in production/ growth of red blood cells	1.3 mg	Lean meats, yeast, beans, yogurt, cheese, milk, green leafy vegetables

Vitamin B6	Brain function; immune system; red blood cells	1.6 mg	Meats, fish, poultry, beans, eggs, white and sweet potatoes, bananas
Vitamin B12	Central nervous system; metabolism	2 mcg	Clams, shellfish; meats; milk; cheese; eggs
Niacin (B3)	Skin; digestive system; converts food into energy	15 mg	Meats, fish, poultry, nuts, grains
Choline	Memory; muscle; healthy cells	425 mg	Eggs, milk, liver, peanuts, cauliflower
Calcium	Bones; heart; muscles; blood clotting	800–1,200 mg	Milk, yogurt, cheese, salmon, sardines, blackstrap molasses, spinach
Magnesium	Energy; muscles; heart; bone development	280 mg	Nuts, meats, tofu, bananas, apricots, yogurt, grains
Iron	Blood; energy; immune system	15 mg	Fish, organ meat, dried fruit, nuts, eggs, enriched bread

Selenium	Thyroid function; antioxidant	55 mcg	Brazil nuts, fish, shellfish, garlic, eggs, poultry, sunflower seeds, red meat, bread, oatmeal, soy nuts
Zinc	Energy/ metabolism; immune system	12 mg	Oysters, seafood; red meat; poultry; nuts; milk; whole grain breads and cereal; tofu; eggs

These are the recommended daily dietary allowances for women between ages 19 and 50, from the Food and Nutrition Board of the National Academy of Sciences and the National Research Council.

How to Take a Multivitamin

- Consult your doctor; have blood work done to find out exactly what you need, especially if you are pregnant or suspect you might have special needs (such as anemia).
- Check the expiration date to be sure the product is still potent.
- Read the label. Watch out for fillers to avoid added sugars, yeast, starches, or additives in your multivitamin. Look for a multivitamin with levels of minerals and vitamins as close as possible to 100 percent of the daily recommended amount (too much can be as bad as too little).

NUTRITION TIP

Remember to eat a healthy, balanced diet. Vitamin supplements are a safeguard, but they cannot fully replace the benefits of the vitamins and minerals we get from food.

- Whether or not you purchase an all-natural synthetic vitamin brand may not matter, with the exception of folate, according to Mary Ellen Camire, Ph.D., professor of Food Science and Human Nutrition at the University of Maine. Our bodies use and absorb the synthetic version of folate more easily.
- To increase absorption of a multivitamin, take it with food, which will slow its breakdown.
- If you are sensitive to the iron in your multivitamin, you may opt to take your multivitamin at night, allowing you to sleep off any side effects the iron may cause, such as stomach irritation. Be sure to take an iron-enriched vitamin with a glass of orange juice (or any form of vitamin C), to help the absorption of the iron. Multivitamins containing iron should not be taken with dairy products, as this will hinder the iron absorption.
- If your supplement contains calcium, be sure it also contains vitamin D, which is crucial to the absorption of calcium.

The Key: Attaching This Step to Your Current Lifestyle

- Taking a vitamin should be like eating breakfast—you need to do it every day. Keep your supplements by your breakfast table so you don't forget.

- If you find you are too busy first thing in the morning to re-member to take your supplement, you may want to keep your multivitamin on the dining table so you remember to take it at dinnertime.
- The trick is to put your vitamins somewhere you will see them every day. After a few weeks, taking a multivitamin will be like second nature to you, and you will wonder why you never did this before—something so good for you and so simple.
- If you normally take your vitamin at work, make sure you have a second bottle at home for the weekends.
- If you find your own unique way to attach this step to your per-sonal lifestyle, please share your ideas with us on our Web site: www.SimpleStepsProgram.com.

Posture and Breathing

Be Aware of Your Posture and Breathing Every Day

Why Are Our Posture and Breathing Important?

· Look into a full-length mirror and stand tall with good posture. Notice how you look 10 pounds thinner?

· Women who stand up straight are perceived as more intelligent and confident, according to Ernst Beier, Ph.D., professor emeritus at the University of Utah and an expert in nonverbal expression.

· How can we expect our children to have good posture until we correct our own?

· Correct your posture and you will certainly reduce back pain.

· Slouching at the computer causes our shoulder muscles to press on nerves and blood vessels that supply blood to our wrists and hands, which can lead to tingling and numbness in fingers.

· When we slouch, enormous pressure is put on our abdomen, neck, and shoulders, slowing digestion.

· Poor posture can reduce the amount of oxygen flowing to our lungs, muscles, and brain. When our body is aligned properly, muscle tension is released and we are able to breathe without effort. Greater flow of oxygen to your brain due to correct breathing creates better mental clarity, states Susan M. Lark, M.D., coauthor of *The Chemistry of Success.*

- As taking slower, deeper breaths increases oxygen in our bloodstream, it also increases our energy level.
- Shallow chest breathing creates an imbalance in the oxygen–carbon dioxide ratio, which may result in hyperventilation and dizziness.
- The average person achieves peak respiratory function and lung capacity during the mid-twenties. We then lose respiratory function at a rate of 10 to 27 percent for every decade of life thereafter, according to Michael Grant White, breathing development specialist, on www.breathing.com. Improving our lung capacity and breathing habits now helps maintain or even improve our general health in the future.
- Slow, deep breathing brings air to the lowest part of our lungs and exercises our diaphragm, which in turn enhances breathing capacity. Deep breathing relaxes our mind and body, massages internal organs, calms emotions, and induces restful sleep.

How to Improve Your Posture and Breathing

POSTURE

- Awareness is the key to good posture. Think about balance and alignment. Everything must be in alignment so both sides of your body carry an equal amount of weight.
- Walk tall: Stand up straight, lift your chin so that it's parallel with the floor, tuck in your abdomen and buttocks, and relax your shoulders. Your ears should be directly over your shoulders, and your chin should be lifted and tucked in slightly.
- High-heeled-shoe lovers beware: Wearing high-heeled shoes

on a regular basis can pull your entire body out of alignment. As often as possible, wear proper fitting low-heeled shoes.

- To check your posture, stand sideways in front of a full-length mirror. Your back should be in a straight line. Then stand facing the mirror and check to be sure everything is in alignment. Are your ears above your shoulders? Are your shoulders above your hips and even on both sides? Kneecaps should be facing forward and ankles straight.
- Test your posture against a wall. Stand with the back of your head touching the wall and heels six inches from the wall. With your buttocks touching the wall, stick your hand between your lower back and the wall and then between your neck and the

---

WEIGHT LOSS TIP

Oxygen is the key to life. One of the main reasons exercise burns fat is it increases your breathing. An increased oxygen intake from proper breathing has been proven to increase your metabolism. That's right—*increase* your metabolism, which can lead to weight loss. Pam Grout, author of *Jumpstart Your Metabolism*, says most overweight people have faulty, but fixable, metabolisms. Oxygen is the fuel that burns fat. Try some deep belly breathing: Begin practicing by lying down flat on your back and holding a book on your belly. Use deep, slow breaths to raise and lower the book. Once you understand the technique, you can practice this breathing anywhere in any position. Deeper, slower belly breathing will change your body chemistry, thereby changing your metabolism, the rate at which your body burns calories from food.

wall. If your lower back is within an inch or two of the wall, and your neck within two inches, you have good posture.

- Position your spine properly by visualizing a string attached to the top of your head. The string is pulling your head up and body into alignment. Ideal posture creates a straight line from your head to your toes, with your shoulders relaxed.

- At the computer, be sure to sit with your feet flat and comfortable on the floor. Your desk should be at a height that allows your shoulders to be relaxed while you use your computer keyboard.

- The computer monitor on your desk should be 5 to 7 inches below eye level. Looking at a downward angle decreases the stress on your neck, according to Dr. Mark Melhorn, orthopedic surgeon and ergonomics expert.

- Use chairs with good lumbar support. Most workplaces provide ergonomically designed chairs and furniture to prevent work-related injuries. Chairs should support your lower back and have adequate cushioning, allowing you to sit comfortably. Your feet should touch the ground with legs bent at a 90-degree angle.

- According to fitness expert Kathy Smith, the isometrics you are already doing daily may help your posture. Smith recommends strengthening your rhomboideus muscles, located between your shoulder blades, by pinching your shoulder blades together several times a day; hold for a count of five, and repeat ten times.

- Smith also recommends working your spinal erector muscles—the muscles alongside your spine—to improve your posture. Lie facedown on your stomach and lift your right leg and the opposite (left) arm and hold for a count of ten. Do the same lift on the other side and repeat three times daily. These posture-improving isometric exercises can be incorporated into your Simple Step from week two.

- Yoga can help improve your posture by increasing flexibility, toning your muscles, and releasing stress. Practice yoga at home using a videotape or take a class.

BREATHING

· Awareness is the first step to improving your breathing. Your inhalation should be equal to your exhalation.

· It's best to inhale and exhale through your nose. Our noses filter out dust and dirt as well as regulate the balance of oxygen and carbon dioxide in our blood. Additionally, nose breathing warms the air and directs more oxygen to the lower lobes of your lungs.

· For optimal health, breathing should be full and rhythmic using the diaphragm to fill and empty the lungs. The movement of your diaphragm controls your breathing.

BREATHING TIP

Practice this breathing exercise to combat stress and tension: Sit comfortably on the floor or lie flat on your back. Relax your hands by your sides or place them on your rib cage to check your breath. Inhale slowly through your nose, expanding your abdomen first, then your rib cage, and finally your upper chest. Don't hold your breath; make a smooth transition into your exhalation. Slowly exhale, emptying your lungs from top to bottom. Shoulders should remain in the same position—don't slouch or raise them as you breathe. Your inhalation should equal your exhalation; try counting to five when you inhale and again when you exhale to be sure they're even. Repeat five times. Breathing techniques can be done anywhere, anytime, to quiet your mind and calm your responses to stress.

The Key: Attaching This Step to Your Current Lifestyle

- Tape small notes on your steering wheel, computer monitor, mirror, and refrigerator to gently remind you to stand up straight and breathe deeply.
- Remind yourself before getting out of bed each morning of the importance of posture and breathing.
- Each time you get into your car or sit at your desk, do a posture check.
- Keep a pillow handy to place behind the small of your back—one in the car and one at your desk.
- Set your watch or personal computer alarm to ring a few times throughout the day as a reminder to sit up straight and concentrate on breathing. When the alarm sounds, check your alignment and readjust.
- At fifteen minutes past each hour get up from your desk and take a breathing break. Spend two minutes concentrating on your breath. Inhale deeply and slowly, filling your belly with air, and then exhale slowly for the same count.
- If you find your own unique way to attach this step to your personal lifestyle, please share your ideas with us on our Web site: www.SimpleStepsProgram.com.

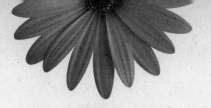

Desktop

Clear Your Desktop and Keep It Organized

Why Should We Organize Our Desktop?

- Whether our desk for business matters is inside or outside of our home, it is important to keep it orderly. It's where we order our lives.
- A clean desktop increases our productivity and improves the quality of our work. A cluttered desk filled with work to be done and papers to be filed causes stress, frustration, and reduced effectiveness.
- An international study by Dr. Peter Honey, an English psychologist and management consultant, documented the best practices of the most effective workers in an information-based work environment. Dr. Honey verified that top performers operated with a clear-desk policy.
- The average desk worker has thirty-six hours of work typically piled on or around his or her desk and wastes about two hours per week looking for things in, on, and around desks, according to Daniel Stamp, founder of Priority Management Systems, a Washington training service specializing in executive produc-

tivity. The real message behind these statistics is that when information piles up, people lose the ability to sort it all out.

How to Organize Your Desktop

- Start by organizing and discarding any useless clutter. Go through all those piles, one at a time. Dump what you no longer need.
- Writer and businessman Larry Hart explains in *Atlanta Business Chronicle* a manageable system to keep desks clean: the "4 D's," simply listed as "Dump, Do, Delegate or Decide." All tasks, and all paper related to the tasks, that now litter your work area can be handled by creating three holding files in one drawer. Label them "mail/correspondence," "projects/miscellaneous," and "reading." Feel free to rename them or add more for your office needs. Gather up all of the paper, including reports, phone message slips, Post-it notes, business cards, notes to yourself, memo pads, and legal pads, and place them in one big pile in the center of your desk. Pull out your daily planner and place it beside the pile. Begin by picking up the first piece of paper and doing one of the following:
  - *Dump* it if it's information you don't need.
  - *Delegate* it to a person who also can get it done.
  - *Do* it yourself right now before you pick up another piece of paper.
  - *Decide* what to do with something you're determined you need to do but cannot take on right now. Make a decision as to when you will actually do the work and note it on the appropriate day in your daily planner. Don't put it all on your to-do list for tomorrow. Spread the work over the next few weeks. Make a note of any due dates in your planner and work accordingly.

- Stay on top of the paper trail that creeps onto your desk by organizing a sensible filing system. Use simplicity. Color-code, alphabetize, or improvise a system that you can remember, and stick to it.

- To help keep clutter off your desktop, have a file drawer within the desk itself. You might even need a second file cabinet within an arm's reach of your desk.

- Treat virtual paperwork (E-mail messages) as you would any other notes. Respond to them and delete them, as they may keep you from tending to items on your desk. You need only 20 percent of what's stored in your mailbox to complete 80 percent of your tasks! Don't be afraid to delete.

- Place all essential items where you can get at them quickly without having to jump up out of your chair. The basics may include computer, phone, appointment book, pens, pencils, stapler, and paper clips.

- To help keep your desktop uncluttered, keep a wastepaper basket close by.

- Install a bulletin board to get some of the smaller reminder notes off of your desk.

- Even if your organizational instincts are intact, it's much harder to control clutter in a cramped space. What if you don't have enough desk space to organize paperwork and supplies? Consider a rolling file cart that can be moved elsewhere if needed but would give you more room to file and store things. Do not use your desktop as a catchall!

The Key: Attaching This Step
to Your Current Lifestyle

- Every afternoon or evening when you are about to leave your desk for the day, take five minutes and go through the paper on your desk. Toss it, file it, or move it elsewhere. It will make a big difference.
- To prevent the paper pile from growing again, apply the "4 D's" to your in-box and daily mail.
- Celebrate TGIF! Every Friday afternoon, before you leave for the weekend, take an extra few minutes and *clean* your desk. Keep a small container of furniture polish or glass cleaner (depending on your desk's surface) in your desk drawer, and sing a happy song as you quickly wipe your desktop.
- Get in the habit of picking up a small inexpensive bouquet of fresh flowers every Monday morning or during Monday's lunch break to brighten up your desktop all week long!
- If you find your own unique way to attach this step to your personal lifestyle, please share your ideas with us on our Web site: www.SimpleStepsProgram.com.

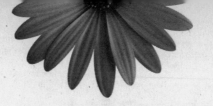

Cleansing Routine

Cleanse and Moisturize Daily

Why Do We Need a Cleansing Routine?

- As we age our skin thins and dries.
- Setting up a proper daily cleansing regimen can help us look younger. We need to keep our skin hydrated and clean to help protect it.
- A proper cleansing routine frees our pores of makeup, dust, and dirt.
- Keeping our face and body clean and soft simply makes us feel good.
- A glowing complexion helps boost our self-confidence.
- Clean and moisturized skin will make us feel refreshed when we are tired or sleep deprived.

How to Cleanse and Moisturize
from Head to Toe

BODY

- In the summer months you should apply an entire shot glass full of sunscreen lotion—that should be reapplied every two to two and a half hours—to all areas of your skin exposed to the sun. Replace old bottles of sunscreen every year, as they lose their effectiveness when past their expiration. Typically lotions last about one year from the date of purchase.
- Use a humidifier in your bedroom during the dry fall and winter months to help moisturize your skin.
- As discussed in our Simple Steps groups, hair conditioner can serve as a useful backup product for moisturizing. Try using hair conditioner as a shaving cream for soft and smooth legs.
- Wash with a loofah sponge to exfoliate your body.
- Use your favorite bath oil, or try this moisturizing bath: Pour a few tablespoons of lemon juice along with ½ cup of baby oil and soak. The lemons will exfoliate while the baby oil will moisturize. Moisturize again with lotion afterwards.
- Use lotion within three minutes of your shower to lock in the moisture before your pores close.

HAIR

- To wash excessive buildup from your hair, use a few tablespoons of baking soda mixed with a cup of water and rinse. Use as needed, once a week if you use a lot of spray, gel, or mousse, or once a month if you don't use a lot of hair products or if you use the same shampoo consistently.

FACE

- Every other day, according to your skin type, you can use a mild and gentle scrub (like oatmeal or apricot) to remove excess dead skin and dirt.

- If you have sensitive skin, be sure to choose fragrance-free and sensitive-skin products.

- Always use cool to warm water when cleansing your skin, as hot water can dry out your skin by washing away your body's natural oils.

- Some women recommend placing a washcloth under warm water and then over your face for a full thirty seconds before you apply a moisturizer. The dampness on your face helps lock in moisture.

- After cleansing and before moisturizing, bring your skin to its natural pH level with a skin toner.

- Use a daily moisturizer specially formulated for use on your face. Use a moisturizer with an SPF of 15 that protects against both UVA and UVB (we all know what the sun can do to our looks!). If you plan on spending the day out in the sun, be sure to increase the SPF by using a sunscreen on your exposed skin. Wear a wide-brimmed hat while doing outside chores, such as gardening.

- Use a lighter moisturizer in the summer because the warmer weather brings out the natural oils in your skin and you sweat more. Use a heavier hydrating cream in the colder, dryer weather because cold weather pulls the moisture out of your skin and it needs to be replaced.

- Some women enjoy a facial mask. Choose a mask according to your skin type. They're good for exfoliating, cleaning out your pores, and rehydrating your skin. Home masks can be used

once a week or once a month, whenever you feel the need to
rejuvenate your skin.

- If you can, treat yourself to a professional facial *at least* once a
year. If you treat yourself only once a year, go in the fall. Summer sun makes your face more susceptible to breakouts and
clogged pores, and a fall cleaning will get your face back into
shape.
- For a home facial, place your face over steaming hot water for
about ten minutes and put a towel over your head and neck to
keep the steam in. When the ten minutes are up, use your usual
cleanser, and then put a mask on for the recommended time.
Once you've removed the mask, use a toner or witch hazel (a
natural astringent) before putting on your moisturizer.
- Apply lip balm or your favorite moisturizing lipstick to keep
your lips from drying out throughout the day. Lips get
sunburned, too!
- Ingredients to look for when purchasing products for antiaging:
alpha hydroxy acid, vitamin C, vitamin A or Retin-A (the most
powerful for those fine lines), vitamin E, Q-10, and antioxidants.
- You don't have to spend a fortune for the cleanser/toner/mois-
turizer that works for you. Read the label to see if it contains
what you are looking for.
- Stop scratching and picking at your face. Scratching dry skin
can cause irritation. Use a skin care product for extra-dry skin
and moisturize the problem away.

HANDS

- Wash your hands thoroughly throughout the day. Lather up for
at least twenty seconds with soap and cool water. (Remember,
hot water can dry out your skin.)
- Keep a pump bottle of moisturizer by your kitchen and bath-

room sinks. After every wash, moisturize your hands. While you're moisturizing, don't forget about your elbows.

FEET

- Use a pumice stone or a foot file after taking a bath or shower to fight calluses on the bottoms of your feet and heels.
- Give yourself a treat: Before going to bed, apply to your feet a heavy coat of petroleum-based lotion (or a foot lotion) and put on a clean pair of white cotton gym socks. When you wake up, your feet will feel smooth and soft.
- Once a week, soak your feet in warm water and shower gel for ten minutes. Exfoliate with a pumice stone or a foot file. Rinse well, apply olive oil to toenails, and gently push back cuticles. Dry and apply cream.

The Key: Attaching This Step to Your Current Lifestyle

- Keep your moisturizing supplies near your toothbrush. Every morning do your cleansing ritual, and then apply a day cream.
- Always carry hand and facial moisturizing creams in your purse so that every time you wash your hands or feel a bit dry you will have it available.
- Every time you wash your hands, sing a song. Sing a favorite tune to ensure you're washing thoroughly—such as "Twinkle, Twinkle, Little Star."
- Every Sunday night, perform a full cleansing and moisturizing routine. Even if you can't keep up with it during the week, you'll feel better if you consistently do it once a week.
- If you find your own unique way to attach this step to your personal lifestyle, please share your ideas with us on our Web site: www.SimpleStepsProgram.com.

Sharing

Debbie Rediscovers Her Self-esteem
As Simple Steps Helps
Her Look and Feel Younger!

Debbie admits that prior to embarking on her Simple Steps journey, life was not that simple. In fact, it was quite chaotic. Her husband, a professional chef, worked long night hours at the restaurant. Evenings were hers alone to raise her two active young boys. Her full-time job during the day had become so dreadful that she despised going to work. And she not only felt older than her years; she realized that she had started *looking* older.

When did this begin? It seemed like just a moment in time ago she had met this romantic man from Italy. She was young and vibrant and lucky enough to be able to travel the world. She loved life and loved this handsome man she would come to marry. She and Antonio were blessed with two beautiful boys when they were in their early forties. Now it seemed Debbie's life was complete. So why didn't she feel fulfilled? A little piece of something seemed to be missing, and as Debbie searched to find answers, she realized that she was missing a piece of herself.

Debbie had hit her highest weight. "I gained a whole other person, about a hundred pounds," she recalls. "I was slender all through my twenties and thirties. After having the two boys, I started putting on the weight and stopped paying attention to me. I stopped

exercising. I was overwhelmed by stress at work." Debbie's relationship with her husband became more distant and strained. "I
just felt like I was getting hit with failure from every direction."

Debbie knew a few friends of hers had joined a lifestyle makeover
group called Simple Steps, but she didn't feel motivated enough for
any self-nurturing at that time. She wasn't quite ready to make a
positive commitment to herself. But she watched and listened. She
saw her friends losing weight and gaining control over their lives,
and they all seemed a little bit happier, somehow. They exuded
positive energy, while she began feeling left behind in a dark cloud.
"I couldn't stand myself anymore. I had to do something."

That January, she decided to join, as a New Year's resolution to
start being good to herself. It was time. "Once I told my husband I
was going to start the program, I knew there was no going back."
From the very first day on the Simple Steps program, Debbie knew
this was for her. Her Simple Step that first week included cleaning
out a drawer. Just one drawer. Well, that seemed easy enough for
her, she thought. "Cleaning out that one drawer did it for me," she
remembers. "I could clearly see a tangible connection between
clutter and my emotional eating. It was such a small, easy task, but
it lifted a thousand negative thoughts from my body. It was as
though I was seeing that my focus had to be shifted. I had to chan-
nel my energies, good or bad, into something constructive. And
wow! How delighted I felt when my kitchen junk drawer was clean
at last! It's empowering! I couldn't believe it!"

Debbie energetically embraced all the Simple Steps assignments after that. They worked. They were manageable. Even with a
busy home and a stressful career, she incorporated each week's
steps into her life. By the second week, Debbie's family and friends
started to see her enthusiasm. "It started switching my whole mood
around. By knowing that I could now take control over small things

in my life, like drinking water and organizing my home, I knew I could handle bigger things."

During the next ten weeks, Debbie lost 25 pounds. Her husband became fascinated with the Simple Steps program and what she was doing. He saw the results and gave her much-needed support to stick with it. Their relationship improved. Though things were still stressful at work, even her coworkers noticed Debbie's new positive attitude. She looked healthier and more youthful. The headaches went away. After years of Debbie's asking and being turned down for a promotion, her boss told her he'd noticed a difference in her and offered her a management position.

"I've learned not to put myself last," says Debbie. "I don't feel guilty anymore for spending time gardening, which is my passion and serenity time. I also found out that support from other women was critical for me. I needed other people cheering me on, keeping me from dwelling on the negatives."

In 2001, Debbie's inspirational story was able to reach millions when she appeared on *The Oprah Winfrey Show* with several other Simple Steps participants, as proof positive that we all can take back control of our life, especially with the camaraderie and guidance of group support.

She has since left her job with plans for starting her own business with her husband. Debbie now facilitates Simple Steps workshops and continues to lead a healthy, happy, and productive life.

Congratulations!

You've now mastered the following Simple Steps. Read them aloud as a positive affirmation. Make them a habit and keep them up as part of your new lifestyle.

I am drinking eight cups of water daily

I am walking twenty minutes a day

I am clearing out one drawer/cabinet/closet space every week

I am saving $2 a day (or 1 percent of my weekly salary)

I am keeping a daily food journal

I am squeezing in some isometrics every day

I am maintaining an efficient laundry system

I am following a daily to-do list

I am taking a multivitamin every day

I am aware of my posture and breathing

I am keeping a clear desktop

I am cleansing and moisturizing daily

WEEK FOUR

The Buttercup

Sweet and inviting. A warm,
buttery yellow blossom.
Small but promising. Forever persistent.

Good Fats

Replace Bad Fats with Good Fats Daily

Why Do We Need Good Fats?

- Good fats are natural fats that help keep our cholesterol low and help raise our HDL, or good cholesterol.
- Monounsaturated fats are the best kind of fats to help raise your HDL. Examples of these fats are olive, peanut, sesame, canola, and avocado oils.
- Polyunsaturated fats are also good to raise your HDL. A few of the foods that contain these fats are corn, soybean, safflower, and cold-water-fish oils.
- Essential fatty acids, such as omega-3 and omega-6, increase our oxidation rate, metabolic rate, and energy level. They also help transport bad cholesterol out of our system and help make joint lubricants. A good balance between omega-3 and omega-6 is also healthy for our cardiovascular system. A few of the foods that contain these fats are fish, nuts, and oils.
- Solid fat, such as shortenings, butter, and fat from meats and poultry, are known as the bad fats and raise your LDL, or bad cholesterol. Keep these saturated fats to a minimum.

- Partially hydrogenated or hydrogenated fats, such as those found in snack foods (cookies, crackers, chips) and many margarines, are harmful to our body and could be linked to breast cancer. Read labels and look for margarines that are free of trans-fatty acids and hydrogenation. Dr. Walter C. Willett, chairman of Nutrition at Harvard School of Public Health, has published a report on a fourteen-year study involving eighty-five thousand nurses. It clearly showed that the nurses who consumed the most trans-fatty acids had the highest rate of heart disease.

How to Consume More Good Fats

- The American Heart Association suggests eating less than 30 percent of your calories in fat per day. You should try to consume 9 percent or fewer of your calories in saturated fats.
- Eat cold-water fish at least two times a week, especially mackerel, salmon, trout, sardines, herring, anchovies, and tuna.
- Substitute extra-virgin olive oil (cold pressed) for butter. Pour a little of the oil onto a plate, season it with a fresh herb such as rosemary or basil, and dip your bread. If you're trying to keep your weight down, limit the oil to 1 teaspoon.
- Bake, broil, or grill your foods. Stir-fry meat and vegetables in a nonstick pan with a teaspoon of monounsaturated oil. If you decide to try using a cooking spray, watch out for hydrogenation.
- Try a variety of poly- or monounsaturated fat oils. If you like spicy foods, try hot chili oil or peanut oil in your stir-fry, or walnut oil as a dressing for your next salad. Experiment and be creative.
- Refrigerate nut and seed oils if you don't plan to use them for a

while. They may solidify while in the refrigerator, so if you need to use them, remove them from the refrigerator a half hour or so before you eat, and shake thoroughly before pouring.

· Polyunsaturated fats (corn, soybean, safflower oils) need to be refrigerated and should not be used with high heat or they can become dangerous to your health.

· Add flaxseed to your cereal each morning. This will add omega-6 fatty acids to your diet.

· Substitute skim milk for whole milk. If you don't like the taste, start with 2 percent fat milk and work your way down to 1 percent or nonfat.

· You can also substitute reduced-fat cheese for regular cheese, reduced sour cream for regular sour cream, and so forth.

· If you like gravy, use a fat separator pouring device, which will automatically hold the fat while you pour the gravy.

· Blot the top of your pizza with a paper towel to remove excess grease and fat. Better yet, try cheese-free pizza.

· Read your labels. Watch for ingredients that contain partially hydrogenated and saturated fats, such as palm and palm kernel oils.

· Get your family involved. If your children go to the grocery store with you, have them help you read the labels at the store and let you know if there are any bad fats in the ingredients.

The Key: Attaching This Step to Your Current Lifestyle

· Make Tuesday and Friday fish days and try some new and tempting recipes.

· To keep your kitchen sweet smelling while cooking fish, put water in a small cooking pot and boil orange peels, clove, or cinnamon sticks at a low temperature. Or simply light your favorite scented candle.

- While grocery shopping, carry a cheat sheet of good fats versus bad fats until you know the difference.
- If you run an errand near a fish market, make it a point to stop in and buy fresh seafood.
- When out to dinner, order a seafood meal (baked, poached, steamed, or grilled) and ask the waiter to hold the butter and/or oil!
- Go through your food journal and highlight bad-fat foods. Plan good-fat replacements for next week.
- Go through your favorite recipes and change bad fats to good fats (olive oil instead of butter, or low-fat cream cheese instead of regular, for example).
- If you find your own unique way to attach this step to your personal lifestyle, please share your ideas with us on our Web site: www.SimpleStepsProgram.com.

Kitchen Dancing

Bring On the Music! Dance to One Song Every Day

Why Should We Dance to Music Every Day?

- Along with its aerobic benefits, kicking up your heels to music allows for physical expression and old-fashioned fun. Dancing is an easy exercise that doesn't require any special equipment. Even if we don't have a radio or CD player in a particular room, we can sing our own tunes!
- Dancing or even just moving to the beat of music is a great, fun combination of two healthy habits: exercising and bringing music into our life.
- Dancing can increase our body's flexibility, gently toning and shaping us.
- Music lifts our heart and soul, and listening to it is a great way to de-stress.
- We have found that people who work out to music may actually work harder without realizing it, and burn more calories, because the music distracts them and makes the exercise seem easier.
- Music can have a profound effect on our emotions. If we're feeling down, we should put on some of our favorite upbeat

songs. Sing along and dance around the kitchen or living room to release our emotions.

- Studies have found music therapy as effective as an analgesic (pain reliever) in increasing pain tolerance and as a relaxant and anxiety reducer for infants and children, as well as for patients with burns, cancer, Alzheimer's, cerebral palsy, stroke, brain injury, or Parkinson's disease, according to the National Institutes of Health in February 1999.

How to Kitchen Dance

- Kitchen dancing is really just dancing at home . . . during the day, in the evening, anytime. You can do it in your bedroom, the family room, the dining room, or even the kitchen!
- You don't have to dance like a pro. In the privacy of your own home, just turn on the tunes and start dancing! Don't worry— no one is watching.
- Tap your toes, sway your hips, snap your fingers, and bop your head to the beat. There is simply no right or wrong way to move. Just get moving and start burning those calories and working off unneeded stress.
- The goal is to dance for at least five minutes a day. But longer is better.
- Practice in front of a mirror if you want to see how a particular dance step looks.
- If you prefer having a dance partner, grab your spouse or swing around your toddler. Hey, you can even dance with your kitchen mop if you want . . . that's the fun part of this exercise—you can do what you want.
- If this step is hard for you at first, don't skip it. Force yourself

to dance to one song a day. You'll be surprised by how quickly it gets to be easy and fun!

The Key: Attaching This Step to Your Current Lifestyle

- Every evening while you're preparing dinner, turn off the TV. Get into the habit of turning on the radio or putting on a favorite CD and dancing in the kitchen. Glide or tap your way around from the refrigerator to the oven, to the sink, back to the fridge, and so on.
- It's so easy to put dancing into your daily routine. Every time you run up and down the stairs, for example, sing a song and wiggle those hips.
- Keep the music on when you're doing other chores, like laundry and drawer de-cluttering. Tap your feet, wiggle your shoulders, and take a full-fledged dance break whenever you need it.
- Try dancing on the balls of your feet like a ballerina to music as you carry your laundry basket to the laundry room.
- Dancing with your family can be a great new tradition to start. Get everyone together for ten minutes of dancing before dinner. It will distract everyone from the predinner munchies and fussiness.
- If you find your own unique way to attach this step to your personal lifestyle, please share your ideas with us on our Web site: www.SimpleStepsProgram.com.

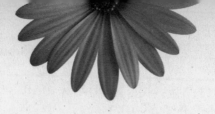

Refrigerator and Pantry

Clean Out Your Fridge and Pantry—Maintain Daily

Why Should We Clean Out Our Fridge and Pantry?

- We will be promoting good health. Having clean and organized food storage spaces helps us keep track of how long we've had food, so we can get spoiled items out of our fridge before someone eats them by mistake or they cause a big stink (literally)!
- We will be able to find what we're looking for. An organized refrigerator means being consistent about where we put different kinds of food.
- Having an organized refrigerator and pantry can help us save money because we won't buy things that we already have, hidden in back shelves or drawers.

How to Clean and Organize the Fridge and Pantry

CLEAN THE REFRIGERATOR

- The best time to clean the refrigerator is the day before your garbage is picked up and the day before you go food shopping and fill the fridge to the brim.
- Begin by emptying everything out of the refrigerator. Yes, milk, juice, eggs, everything. Seeing these items out on your counters should inspire you to work quickly. If you're worried about particularly temperature-sensitive foods spoiling, you can place these items in a temporary cooler.
- Clean all the shelves and drawers. Most refrigerators can be cleaned with a damp towel, but check your refrigerator manual for specific cleaning suggestions.
- After you wash the shelves and drawers, apply just a drop of glycerin on a soft cloth and wipe off the shelves and drawers. The glycerin will help prevent any future spills from sticking to the shelves. You can find glycerin in the hand cream section of any drugstore.
- If your refrigerator is in need of major cleaning, take the shelves and drawers out completely and wash them in the sink or dishwasher with warm water and mild soap or detergent. Rinse and dry thoroughly before replacing.
- Wash the refrigerator door seal with water and mild detergent. Rinse and dry. Apply a thin coat of petroleum jelly to keep the seal pliable.
- Vacuum the condenser coils and vents at the bottom of the fridge or in the back a few times per year (more often if you have pets). Remove and wash the drip pan if possible.
- To keep off the dust that collects on the top of your refrigerator,

dampen and cover the entire top with a sheet of plastic wrap or wax paper. Occasionally discard and replace.

- Don't forget to wipe down the outside of the fridge to remove sticky fingerprints from the door handles.
- Set your refrigerator at 40 degrees Fahrenheit or lower to keep foods from spoiling too quickly.
- Change your refrigerator box of baking soda every month, or simply use a cotton ball dipped in essence of lemon oil placed on the back of a shelf to help keep odors away and leave a clean scent.
- With a warm, wet cloth, wipe off bottle tops and bottoms (of ketchup, maple syrup, etc.).

ORGANIZE THE REFRIGERATOR

- Keep your water bottles on the top shelf in front. (Remember to drink your eight glasses daily.) Your milk and orange juice should also earn a front spot for convenience.
- Use the second shelf as your snack shelf for yogurts, fresh berries, and salsa.
- Think meal ideas: Maybe use the third shelf for easy meal fixings. Keep your wrapped leftover chicken next to a tomato and salad greens for a quick salad, or low-fat cheese and sauce next to a container of precooked pasta.
- Use your refrigerator door to store fresh herbs, flavorings, and condiments. Put fat-free dressings next to fresh garlic and basil for quick toppings.
- Store eggs in their cartons, not on the refrigerator egg shelf. This helps prevent the eggs from absorbing the flavor of other foods while preserving their own moisture.
- Remember that most leftover food lasts only two to five days in the fridge. Keep leftovers securely wrapped at the front of the

shelf so you will notice them, and toss them out if not eaten. As far as food freshness, remember, when in doubt, throw it out!

- Special produce bags, such as Evert-Fresh and PEAKfresh bag brands, are available in most supermarkets in the produce section. They claim to keep produce fresh for up to three weeks!

- Thaw frozen foods in covered containers in your refrigerator, instead of on the counter at room temperature. In case children or other family members move the shelf items or open the containers to peek in, always place defrosting meats on the *bottom* shelf, so drips cannot contaminate foods below.

- Having an organized refrigerator means cleaning, cutting, preparing, and displaying produce for healthy quick-grab snacks.

- Keep your fridge organized after you've cleaned it. Daily maintenance means always putting foods back into their proper place.

CHATTER TIME

Gretchen, a mother of three preschool-aged children, told her Simple Steps group that she created a kids' healthy-snack shelf in her fridge. Prefilled juice sip cups, small water bottles, a bowl of washed grapes, and peeled baby carrots were all arranged on a lower shelf so that her young children could help themselves to healthy snacks.

THE FREEZER

- Thoroughly clean your freezer this week, too.
- Freezers are most efficient when they are full, so keep yours well stocked, but leave room between each item so that the chilled air can circulate.
- If needed, defrost your freezer. Spray a light coating of cooking oil on the freezer's interior walls. It will keep icy buildup away.
- Set your freezer temperature between 0 and 5 degrees Fahrenheit.
- To preserve freshness and inhibit frost buildup on food in the freezer, squeeze all the air from the plastic bags in which you store food, then quickly seal the bags.
- Buy clear, freezer-safe stackable containers and label them with the date stored so you can use the oldest packages first.
- Arrange containers so it's easy to reach the ones you use most frequently.
- Categorize each freezer shelf by like items so you can find things quickly. Store frozen vegetables on one shelf, beef products on another, poultry or seafood on another, and so on.

THE FOOD PANTRY

- Start by clearing out your entire food pantry.
- Wipe down all shelves. Sweep and vacuum if you have a walk-in pantry.
- Check expiration dates on cereal boxes and other items that you haven't used in a while.
- Invest in stackable see-through containers. Use them for everything from pastas and rice to snacks and cereal. These containers not only look neat and organized but they also protect your food from pests and preserve the food's longevity. This will help you inspect the condition of all your dry foods as

well. Make sure the containers are tightly sealed, and place a
bay leaf in each one to keep insects away from flour, pastas, and
beans.

· To help prevent certain household pests, try not to keep foods
in low-level kitchen areas, such as shelf space below counters.

WEIGHT LOSS TIP

Eliminate your trigger food. If you have a problem food that
tempts you off your diet, such as chocolate chip cookies or potato chips, instead of hiding them on the top shelf of your pantry
in a brown bag (who are you kidding?), the best solution is to
simply not have the food in your pantry whatsoever. Chances
are the others in your household do not need that food either!

· Keep in your pantry a shopping list with a pencil attached to it.
Make note of when you finish an item and need to purchase
more.

· Hang a corkboard square on the inside of your pantry door to
hold recipes, labels of foods you want to remember, and grocery lists.

· If you have room in your pantry, buy regularly used items in
bulk to save money.

SAFE FOOD STORAGE AT HOME

Examples based on both perishable and nonperishable foods, all stored tightly sealed.

IN THE REFRIGERATOR

Eggs (average shelf life after sell-by date)	2 weeks
Butter/margarine	2 weeks
Luncheon meats	7 days
Milk (after sell-by date)	5–7 days
Fresh meat (poultry, roasts, steaks, chops)	3–5 days
Soft cheeses (cottage, ricotta)	3 days
Cut-up uncooked poultry	3 days
Cooked poultry or meats	1–2 days
Fresh fish (stored in fridge, on ice and wrapped)	1–2 days

IN THE FREEZER

Frozen seafood	3–6 months
Ground beef and lamb	3–4 months
Precooked combo dinners	3–4 months
Ground pork	1–3 months
Ham, bacon, luncheon meats	2–3 weeks

IN THE PANTRY

Canned fruits and fruit juices	18–36 months
Canned vegetables	8–12 months
Canned acidic vegetables (tomatoes, sauerkraut)	12 months
Breakfast cereals (unopened)	6–18 months

Macaroni/spaghetti, etc.	6–9 months
Mayonnaise and salad dressings (unopened)	2 months
Cookies and crackers (unopened)	1–6 months
Ground coffee (not vacuum-packed)	2 weeks

Applied Foodservice Sanitation, 2nd ed., D.C. Heath Company and National Institute for the Food Service Industry.

The Key: Attaching This Step to Your Current Lifestyle

- Get in the habit of putting items back where they belong in your fridge, freezer, or pantry. Use a label gun to mark the purpose of a particular shelf or drawer.
- When wiping down your kitchen counters every morning or evening before you go to bed, wipe down the outside of your fridge as well.
- Every time you reach for a water bottle in the fridge, take a moment and double-check the organization of the foods.
- When you open your pantry to retrieve a food item, double-check its organization as well. Always put foods back in the same location you found them.
- In your pantry, place easy-to-grab healthy snacks at eye level (whole wheat pretzels, applesauce, soy nuts).
- When you plan to grocery shop, schedule in an extra fifteen to thirty minutes so you won't feel rushed and end up cramming everything into the refrigerator when you unpack your grocery bags. This will help you start the week off more organized and relaxed.

- Stick a note on your refrigerator that says "What you are looking for is NOT in here!" to help curb mindless eating.
- If you find your own unique way to attach this step to your personal lifestyle, please share your ideas with us on our Web site: www.SimpleStepsProgram.com.

Dental Hygiene

Clean and Floss Your Teeth Twice Daily

Why Do We Need to Clean and Floss Our Teeth Daily?

- Brushing and flossing our teeth brightens our smile, enhances our self-confidence, and helps prevent tooth decay, bacterial infections, and tooth loss.
- Bacteria removed within twenty-four hours of settling on a tooth's surface have less chance to damage teeth or cause gum disease.
- Brushing can do more than clean our teeth and freshen our breath. According to a University of Minnesota study, proper brushing can help prevent blood clots, heart attacks, and strokes. Research revealed that bacterial deposits accumulated on teeth due to lack of regular brushing can find their way into the bloodstream and help form blood clots.
- Brushing without flossing is like washing only 80 percent of your body. The other 20 percent remains dirty.
- Avoid gum disease by flossing at least once daily to strengthen gums and remove bacteria. Flossing prevents cavities and tooth decay in areas where a toothbrush cannot reach.

• Scheduling regular checkups with our dentist is also important for our teeth as well as our health.

CHATTER TIME

After Susan received her Simple Step assignment to practice good oral hygiene, she shared the following story: When she had her dental cleaning that week, her dentist reviewed the proper techniques for brushing and flossing. Susan admitted to her dentist she did not floss and thought it unnecessary because her teeth had plenty of space to brush between them. The dentist stressed the importance of flossing, and Susan asked whether it was adequate to floss only her back teeth because they were closer together. Her dentist smiled and answered, *"Only floss the teeth you want to keep."*

How to Practice Good Oral Hygiene

• The American Dental Association (ADA) recommends brushing two times a day with fluoride toothpaste, flossing in between teeth at least once a day, and using a fluoride rinse.
• Buy a toothbrush with a small head for easier access to all parts of your mouth, teeth, and gums. Be sure it has soft bristles with rounded ends so you don't injure your gums.
• Use any toothpaste with fluoride as long as it carries the ADA seal of acceptance.
• Brushing should take at least two minutes, according to Dr. Anthony Vocaturo, an official dentist for the Miss USA Pageant.

Dr. Vocaturo also stresses the importance of brushing your
tongue and the roof of your mouth.

- The two most important times to brush your teeth are after
breakfast and before bed. That's when bacterial residue is at its
highest, suggests Dr. Julie Barna, family dentist in Lewisburg,
Pennsylvania, and a Master at the Academy of General Den-
tistry. If you want to brush during the day but can't, chew sugarless gum and rinse your mouth with water.

- Change your toothbrush every three months. The seasonal
change—a new toothbrush with every season—is an easy rule to
remember. Change your toothbrush immediately after you
recover from any illness, even if it's just a winter cold.

- Store your toothbrush in an open, dry place, not in a plastic
case where it's easier for bacteria to grow.

- Don't share your toothbrush with anyone. Your toothbrush can
harbor bacteria and viruses. Some flu germs can survive on a
toothbrush for up to twenty-four hours.

- Soaking your toothbrush in antibacterial rinse such as Listerine
can help prevent bacterial growth.

- Dental floss comes in various forms. Products such as Glide
dental floss are recommended if your teeth are close together
because the coated Teflon floss won't fray. Dental tapes
work best for those with widely spaced teeth or bridgework.
Ask your dentist to help you find the product that works best
for you.

- To properly floss, the American Dental Association suggests,
wrap the floss around each tooth and gently rub side to side,
moving the floss up and down the entire tooth. Proper flossing
takes practice.

- Unwaxed floss squeaks when you have thoroughly cleaned between your teeth.

- Rinsing or brushing after flossing will help remove any plaque dislodged during flossing.
- Brush and rinse with warm water if you have sensitive teeth.
- In addition to daily cleaning, visit the dentist at least biannually to have your teeth professionally cleaned.

The Key: Attaching This Step to Your Current Lifestyle

- Brush and floss your teeth at the same time every day. Establish a consistent daily routine when brushing your teeth. Store the necessary items—toothbrush, toothpaste, floss, and rinse—together so you don't skip or forget one.
- Keep dental floss containers in convenient places throughout your home (for example, on your nightstand; in the kitchen, where you do most of your eating; in your car; and on your office desk).
- While at the dentist's office, schedule your *next* cleaning appointment immediately after having your teeth cleaned. If you don't, you may forget and end up waiting longer than six months before the next visit.
- Buy more than one toothbrush and keep an extra at work. Brushing your teeth at work without toothpaste is more effective than not brushing at all. Of course, brush at home in the morning and evening with fluoride toothpaste for cavity prevention.
- Keep dental mints (such as Biotene mints) or dental chewing gum (such as Trident Advantage or Aquafresh Dental Gum) in your purse for times when you cannot brush or floss after eating. According to an ADA news release dated July 2000, chewing gum containing xylitol can be helpful in controlling tooth

decay; xylitol (made from the bark of birch trees) temporarily neutralizes bacteria that cause tooth decay.

- When you are away from home and can't brush or floss, rinse your mouth with water to help loosen food particles from between teeth.
- We never forget to have our children brush, so brush every morning and evening with the kids.
- If you find your own unique way to attach this step to your personal lifestyle, please share your ideas with us on our Web site: www.SimpleStepsProgram.com.

Sharing

Healthier Cooking and Better
Organization Changed Sarah's Life!

Give Sarah two minutes and she can put her hands on the Christmas card list, the swim club schedule, or the school calendar. It's one result of her newly organized life after ten weeks on the Simple Steps program. It's also a life that's 17 pounds lighter. "I never thought about it before I joined the group. It's true, this whole idea—when your life is in order, your body will follow. When my life is in order, I can control my weight."

Sarah is the wife of a doctor and the mother of two young girls. She says every time she looked for something, it used to take her at least twenty minutes to find it, if she found it at all. The disorganization drained her energy and made her feel stressed. When she started on her Simple Steps journey, it gave her new direction. The steps made sense to her. They were simple and easy to fit into her daily lifestyle, and yet they seemed to have tremendous impact on her. Other women in her group shared tips on things like household organization and better time management. "I now believe there really is a place for everything," she says. "We get complacent about keeping our life in order. I've come to realize that everything looks worse in your life if nothing is organized. If you keep track of things on a daily basis, then you don't feel like everything is falling down around you."

Sarah went on a mission to get her house completely organized once and for all. She created a system of binders that she keeps under her kitchen sink to hold all the paper clutter that comes into the house. "As soon as a note comes home from school, it goes into the school binder," she says, "and when the mail comes, I now sort it and throw out the junk, right away."

But perhaps even more than helping Sarah become an organized person, the program also taught her how to start taking care of herself and to put herself first sometimes. "I had to find time to exercise, which isn't easy with two small children. Normally, if I had a baby-sitter, I'd use those hours to go to the grocery store and run errands. Now I use that time to go for a run or ride my bike. When I exercise," she insists, "I feel so much better afterward. All the things that might have seemed overwhelming are suddenly not so overwhelming after I've worked out. To me, exercise is a real time of solace and a kind of relaxation."

Everything in her life began to come together. It was as though her life had been a big jigsaw puzzle of loose pieces, and now she was finally putting the pieces into place. When Sarah started organizing her home, her time management improved, and so she began scheduling time to work out. When Sarah exercised, she found that she automatically started paying more attention to what she was eating.

Simple Steps gave her the guidance she needed for healthy eating. She was ready for change. She learned the difference between good fats and bad fats, and about better food choices in general. Many women in her group shared light and nutritious recipes that tasted great. Sarah was inspired. She started cooking healthier. "I remember when I used to grab whatever was quick and available, like crackers and junk. Now I keep a lot of fresh vegetables and fruits in the house and I'm really watching portion sizes." Sarah works at keeping her refrigerator and food pantry well stocked with healthy foods, but she knows that sometimes she still has to will herself away from munching. "I also learned from the program that I'm not always hungry when I nibble," admits Sarah, who realized she had been eating for the wrong reasons. "Sometimes when I have the urge to eat now, I just pick myself up and do something else, like go outside and play with the kids or organize a drawer. I just get myself out of the kitchen."

Sarah's doctor husband has also become a big supporter of Simple Steps. One day Tom, the husband of Simple Steps coauthor Beverly, went in for his annual checkup. Tom was surprised when his doctor came in and exclaimed, "I love your wife! Because of the Simple Steps program, my wife, Sarah, is cooking better, and even I lost twenty-five pounds!" The ripple effect. When Sarah started cooking healthier, everyone in the family started eating better and reaping the benefits.

"It's all interconnected," Sarah concludes. "Everyone who sees me knows that I have a much better outlook on life now. When I finally got control over things that were bothering me, all other aspects of my life became easier. My clothes fit better, and I've gotten rid of the extra baggage . . . not just on my body, but in my life."

Congratulations!

You've now mastered the following Simple Steps. Read them aloud as a positive affirmation. Make them a habit and keep them up as part of your new lifestyle.

I am drinking eight cups of water daily

I am walking twenty minutes a day

I am clearing out one drawer/cabinet/closet space every week

I am saving $2 a day (or 1 percent of my weekly salary)

I am keeping a daily food journal

I am squeezing in some isometrics every day

I am maintaining an efficient laundry system

I am following a daily to-do list

I am taking a multivitamin every day

I am aware of my posture and breathing

I am keeping a clear desktop

I am cleansing and moisturizing daily

I am replacing bad fats with good fats

I am dancing to at least one song every day

I am maintaining a clean and healthy refrigerator and pantry

I am cleaning and flossing my teeth twice daily

Lavender

Calming and fragrant.
Gentle and soothing is her soul.

Caffeine Cutback

Reduce Caffeine Intake

Why Should We Cut Back On Caffeine?

- Caffeine is a stimulant that in small amounts may produce alertness and faster reaction time in some people; however, overdoses can cause headaches, trembling, an abnormally fast heart rate, an upset stomach, nervousness, sleeplessness, irritability, and diarrhea.
- Caffeine can stiffen arteries and increase the risk of stroke and heart failure. Drinking excessive amounts of caffeine can cause arrhythmia, where our heart skips beats. Caffeine increases our heart rate and our blood pressure.
- Caffeine acts as a diuretic, which may leave us dehydrated.
- Caffeine increases urinary excretion of calcium, states Dr. J. C. Gallagher, director of the Bone Metabolism Unit at Creighton University in Nebraska, and therefore this calcium loss from our body can lead to osteoporosis.
- Caffeinated drinks can aggravate irritable bowel syndrome, or IBS, and can lead to excessive cramps, according to Blue Cross and Blue Shield at www.blueprint.bluecrossmn.com.

- Francine Grodstein, Ph.D., an epidemiologist at Harvard School of Public Health, found that women who drank more than two cups of caffeinated coffee or tea, or more than four cans of cola per day, had a greater risk of infertility problems. Caffeine constricts blood flow, which could affect the fallopian tubes and stimulate estrogen production, which may lead to endometriosis.

How to Cut Back on Caffeine

- Start by paying attention to your caffeine intake, being aware of your consumption.
- If you feel the need for a second cup of coffee, try drinking a decaffeinated coffee, which comes in many different flavors. Find a flavor you enjoy.
- Cut back slowly. Start by limiting yourself to drinking two cups of coffee or two cans of soda per day. Or set a time limit, such as not drinking coffee after two P.M. The following week, finish coffee before noon.
- Caffeine withdrawal can involve some side effects, including headaches and difficulty concentrating. If you are a heavy caffeine drinker, gradually reduce your consumption from multiple cups of coffee or other highly caffeinated beverages to just a few and then just one. Eventually you may even want to replace that one cup with a single decaf. (Many women report that once they adjust to a lower level of caffeine in their systems, a single decaf can wake them up just as much as ten cups of coffee used to.) Someday, you may even be able to replace that single decaf with herbal tea. Once you've kicked the caffeine habit, you'll be amazed to discover how alert you are naturally when you wake up in the morning.

· If you need your morning coffee, go ahead and enjoy it; just stop there. A single cup of coffee can boost your energy level for up to six hours, report researchers from the Massachusetts Institute of Technology.

CAFFEINE FOUND IN DRINKS

CAFFEINE IN A 7-OZ CUP OF COFFEE/TEA:

Drip	115–175 mg
Brewed	80–135 mg
Instant	65–100 mg
Espresso (1 oz)	50 mg
Decaf, brewed	3–4 mg
Decaf, instant	2–3 mg
Tea, brewed	40–60 mg
Tea, instant	30 mg

CAFFEINE IN A 12-OZ CAN OF SODA:

Jolt	80 mg
Mountain Dew	55 mg
Mello Yello	52.8 mg
Coca-Cola	46 mg
Sunkist Orange	40 mg
Pepsi	37.2 mg
Canada Dry Cola	30 mg
Canada Dry Diet Cola	1.2 mg
7 UP	0
Sprite	0
Minute Maid Orange	0

CAFFEINE IN OTHER:

NoDoz, max. strength, 1 tablet	200 mg
Excedrin, 2 tablets	130 mg
NoDoz, reg. strength, 1 tablet	100 mg
Anacin, 2 tablets	64 mg
Dannon Coffee Yogurt, 8 oz	45 mg
1.4-oz bar of dark chocolate	28 mg
Chocolate, unsweetened—1 oz, Baker's brand	25 mg
Semi-sweet chocolate—1 oz, Baker's	13 mg
German sweet chocolate—1 oz, Baker's	8 mg
Coffee Nips, 2 pieces	6 mg
1.4-oz bar of milk chocolate	3–10 mg
Chocolate milk—8 oz	2–7 mg
1.4-oz bar of white chocolate	2–4 mg
Stonyfield Farm Cappuccino Yogurt, 8 oz	0 mg

In accordance with data from the National Soft Drink Association

The Key: Attaching This Step to Your Current Lifestyle

· Replace your second daily cup of coffee with a cup of decaf. After a couple of weeks, replace it with herbal tea.
· Instead of drinking a caffeinated soda, try a mineral or seltzer water for something bubbly. For flavor, add a twist of citrus fruit or a splash of your favorite juice.
· Every time you want to have a cup of coffee, do some stretches or deep-breathing exercises.
· If your favorite coffee shop is on your way to work, order a de-

caffeinated coffee or an herbal tea. Better yet, change your driving route.

- The money that you save by not buying extra cups of coffee throughout the day could be added to your rainy-day savings fund, or reward yourself with a manicure, facial, or a new pair of shoes.

CHITCHAT

I never thought I was a big coffee drinker. I would always have my last cup of java before two P.M., which was my rule. I realized that I needed to stop drinking coffee when my face started to become so tense and I had a big crinkle running right through the center of my forehead. I couldn't get it to relax at all; it was a very uncomfortable feeling. If caffeine was doing this to my face, I could imagine what it was doing to the rest of my body! When I first cut back on my caffeine intake, the withdrawal was so powerful I almost started drinking coffee again. But the headaches were gone within a week and so were the tense muscles in my face. I feel much better and currently drink either water or a cup of decaffeinated coffee to start my day.

—Linda McClintock

- Try buying a coffeemaker that brews just two to four cups, so you (and your housemates) can't easily pour too many cups.
- If you find your own unique way to attach this step to your personal lifestyle, please share your ideas with us on our Web site: www.SimpleStepsProgram.com.

Yoga

Practice Fifteen Minutes of Yoga Each Day

Why Should We Practice Yoga?

- Yoga postures (*asanas*) are gentle stretching movements designed to help balance our mind and body. The postures rejuvenate the brain, spine, glands, and internal organs by increasing blood flow and oxygen to these areas.
- Yoga uses movement, breath, posture, relaxation, and meditation to achieve a healthy, vibrant, and balanced approach to life.
- The word *yoga* means to merge, join, or unite. The typical yoga session blends strength, flexibility, and mind/body awareness.
- Yoga is a safe and easy way for all ages to exercise.
- Breathing during yoga (called *pranayama*) is the link between the physical and mental disciplines of yoga. Controlling our breath can bring about beneficial changes for our mind and body.
- Most yoga teachers believe that breathing should be done in and out of our nose because it creates more energy. Nose breathing also filters out dirt and moisturizes and warms in-

coming air, according to Sudha Carolyn Lundeen in an article at www.yogajournal.com.

- Yoga allows us to work to our own individual fitness level, and yoga postures help us become more flexible by stretching and extending our spine. Balance and coordination also improve with yoga.
- Yoga engages and challenges almost every muscle in our body.
- Muscles shorten with age and joints become tight. Yoga restretches and tones muscles while helping relieve stiffness in joints.
- Yoga helps with pain associated with osteoarthritis and carpal tunnel syndrome, according to the February 2000 issue of the journal *Rheumatic Disease Clinics of North America*.
- Yoga postures can stimulate our thyroid gland, which directly affects our metabolism (or the rate at which our body burns fat).
- One hour of yoga burns approximately 244 calories. Doing fifteen minutes will burn approximately 61 calories.
- Our posture can drastically improve with yoga, thereby improving our breathing and concentration because we're in a position that allows our lungs to expand. More oxygen in our blood and to our brain increases our energy and sharpens our focus.
- Through relaxation and proper breathing, yoga releases endorphins from the pleasure center in our brain.
- Yoga encourages self-awareness and mindfulness in everyday life. It is a physical, mental, and spiritual workout.

FIVE-MINUTE YOGA STRESS RELEASE

Why not take five minutes upon returning home after a stressful day to unwind with yoga? Massage therapist Cheryl McKereghan advises the following posture: Lie with your back on the floor and your legs fully extended and raised against a wall. Keep your arms at your sides in a comfortable position. Take a deep breath and then exhale through your nose five times in short, sharp breaths. Repeat to reach a total of ten times. This position will allow blood to drain from your lower legs and ankles, and the breathing will help you to relax and clear your head.

How to Practice Yoga

- To get started, work with a yoga book or video to follow until you are confident practicing the basic postures. You might want to try a class. It is helpful to tune in to the voice of the instructor and concentrate on your breath.
- Ask your family not to interrupt you during your fifteen-minute yoga time. If necessary, place a DO NOT DISTURB sign on the door.
- Practice yoga with an empty stomach. Allow two hours for you to digest any food eaten, and if possible, empty your bowels and bladder before beginning. Bending and stretching during postures can cause internal pressure on some of your organs, so having a full stomach, bowels, or bladder could cause discomfort, dizziness, or nausea.
- Dress comfortably and be sure your clothing does not restrict

your movement. Most people practice yoga with bare feet, not only so they don't slip, but to allow their feet to breathe and feel the exercise.

- Use a blanket, towel, or yoga sticky mat when practicing yoga.
- Light a scented candle and lower the lights to encourage relaxation.
- Yoga movements are done in conjunction with slow, deep breathing. Movements are performed slowly with fluid motions.
- When doing yoga strive for precise, accurate movements. Quality in your postures is more important than quantity.
- Try to alternate postures daily to spice up your routine and to exercise different parts of your body.
- Try more than one yoga class. Call the teacher before starting the class to discuss the benefits you are seeking from yoga. There are several different types of yoga that offer various benefits for flexibility and building muscle strength.

The Key: Attaching This Step to Your Current Lifestyle

- Schedule yoga into your day by writing it in your daily planner or on your to-do list.
- Yoga will become a habit if you practice it daily at the same time. Try practicing your yoga postures first thing in the morning or right before you go to bed. You may even find the calming practice of yoga helps you sleep better.
- Start small if you must. Spend five minutes a day practicing a few favorite yoga postures. Before long, you will feel the benefit and wisely begin spending more time daily practicing yoga.

- Get your children involved. Find a beginners class for kids while you go to your class.
- If you find your own unique way to attach this step to your personal lifestyle, please share your ideas with us on our Web site: www.SimpleStepsProgram.com.

Mail Clutter

SIMPLE STEP 19

Get Rid of the Mail Pile
on Your Counter

Why Should We Get Rid of Our Mail Pile?

- A mail pile is more clutter in our home. Clutter causes stress and distraction.
- With a stack of mail already on our counter, we're more likely to continue the path of disorder. Tomorrow's mail already has an inviting resting place. And the day after that . . .
- A disorganized mail pile can lead to lost and overdue bills. When we get rid of our mail pile through proper organizational filing, we are less likely to lose or misplace these important pieces of mail.
- Magazines can become a big, bottomless pile preventing us from knowing what we have or haven't read.

How to Delete a Mail Pile

- Getting rid of a mail pile means setting up an efficient system for organization.
- Sort through your mail every day, separating and discarding

mail you don't need, as soon as you retrieve mail from your mailbox.

- If you have a large family and a heavy mail volume, consider buying a plastic organizer with a slot to hold the mail for each member of your family. (But keep it out of your tidy kitchen!)
- Only hold the mail *once!* While that stack of envelopes is in your hand, sort through it and tend to each piece of mail immediately. Never set any mail down on your kitchen counter, even as a temporary resting place.
- Open your mail near the garbage can.
- Set up a designated mail zone on a home desk or office area for bills to be paid. Make sure you implement an efficient sorting system, or you will simply be creating another mail pile in your home.
- Remove the outer envelopes from all bills—the pile will be half the size! If you pay bills twice a month, organize them into a desktop sorter with two slots labeled "1st" and "15th." When a bill arrives that you routinely pay on the first of the month, simply file it in the first slot. Use the second slot for bills to be paid on the fifteenth.
- A thirty-one-day sorting system (a desktop organizer with thirty-one slots) allows you to file bills according to the mail-by date. Mail sorting organizers are available at all office supply stores as well as many discount department stores.
- Throw out all junk mail. *Tip:* If it's something important, it should have first-class postage or a label on it.
- Distribute the magazines you're going to read to the places most conducive to doing that, whether that means the magazine rack at your bedside, a bin under the coffee table in the family room, or the magazine rack in the bathroom.
- Old magazines should be recycled or given away every month. Do not hesitate to part with those thick, glossy, expensive mag-

azines. Once you've read them, you've received your money's worth. Recycle them to local elementary schools and hospitals, where they can be used for crafts projects. (You might consider saving a few in a neatly labeled bin to use for your treasure-mapping project in week ten.)

- If you like to save magazine articles, set up a file for them. Organize it by subjects, such as recipes, crafts, or gift ideas, and write down the date on it. If you haven't read the article after a six-month or one-year period, toss if. If you can, try to recycle what you discard.

- If you normally make purchases from a favorite catalog, look through it as soon as it arrives and pull out possible purchase items along with the order form. Put them in your magazine file and discard the rest. If you can't afford it right now, do not save the catalog. Toss it. You can always request a new and updated catalog at a later date or log on to the store's Web site.

- If you are receiving duplicate copies of catalogs, send both labels to the cataloger with one label crossed out.

- Get your name off junk mailing lists! This should reduce the amount of unsolicited mail you receive. Send a postcard or letter asking to have your name removed from all lists. Write to Direct Marketing Association/Mail Preference Service, P.O. Box 9008, Farmington, NY 11735-9008.

The Key: Attaching This Step to Your Current Lifestyle

- When you normally go out to get your mail, get into the habit of swinging by the family's main trash pail in the garage or kitchen, or, even better, the one outside your home. Sort over the trash and toss as much as you can.

CHATTER TIME

A few Simple Steps participants recently decided to band to-gether for de-cluttering their mail. Each of the women set up a magazine basket/bin in her garage (out of sight but within reach). The women agreed to throw in every single magazine or catalog that came into their homes via the mail for one month. At the end of the month they got together with their baskets of collected magazines for a creative and fun girls' night out, ex-changing magazines, flipping through the glossy pages, and cutting out pictures for treasure map sessions they learned about in week ten. *The results:* Each woman was amazed at just how much glossy-paged mail entered her home. All magazines and catalogs had been cleared off counters instantly, and after the women's get-together, they combined their leftover maga-zines and dropped them off at the local recycling center. The women now plan to do this a few times a year.

- During family breakfast or dinner, hand out personal mail to family members and make it a point to tell all of them to check their mail slot and empty it before watching television or hav-ing dessert. By a designated time of evening, the mail sorter should be completely cleared.
- Important outgoing mail should be placed in a hanging file rack near your house keys. Keep an ample supply of postage stamps at your bill-paying station.
- Keep a letter opener handy near your mail-sorting zone.
- If you find your own unique way to attach this step to your per-sonal lifestyle, please share your ideas with us on our Web site: www.SimpleStepsProgram.com.

Daily Serenity Time

Find Ten Minutes of Solitude Every Day

Why Do We Need Daily Serenity Time?

- We need daily serenity time for relaxation and stress relief. We lead overscheduled, overstimulated lives, and we simply need an ample supply of quiet downtime for keeping a comfortable balance in our lives.
- During quiet time, levels of adrenaline (chemical messengers) and cortisol (the primary stress hormone) in our blood decrease, increasing the feeling of calm, notes Eva Stubits of University of Texas Medical School in Houston.
- Serenity time can be soul cleansing.
- Serenity time on a daily basis may help keep some illnesses at bay. Severe chronic stress is now linked as a contributor to four of the leading causes of death in American women: heart disease, cancer, lung disease, and accidents.
- Ten minutes of solitude every day allows us time for our imaginations to run free with creativity.
- Daily serenity time recharges our energy.
- Daily serenity time gives us a quiet moment to reflect on the simple pleasures in our life. It helps connect us again to cher-

ished memories, thoughts, and actions that might have otherwise been missed in a life that goes by at a hundred miles per hour.

· Taking time to de-stress and pamper ourselves every day can make our bodies feel more youthful by as many as thirty years, according to the results of a study conducted by Dr. Michael Roizen of the University of Chicago.

· Daily serenity time is about taking care of us and nurturing our soul. We can only effectively nurture other relationships when our own life is properly nurtured.

· Daily serenity time may be the only quiet time we enjoy during the day. According to many Simple Steps participants, they feel their *job* never ends. Most women run their households seven days of the week, whether they work outside the home or not, with no time off after five p.m. or on the weekends. Simply, every woman needs a quiet and peaceful respite every day.

How to Practice Serenity Time Every Day

· Take a close look at your typical daily schedule. Is there a time of day in which you could carve out ten minutes or so away from everyone?

· Create a comfortable serenity place of your own to retreat to. It might contain a corner bedroom table with a burning candle and a favorite photo displayed, or it might be a comfy family room chair or backyard hammock. Find a small, sunny corner and drift off to a pleasant daydream. Seek out a quiet place that you associate with peace and serenity.

· Set a timer for ten minutes and practice not worrying about anything until it goes off.

· To begin a serenity routine, take a seat, relax, and get comfortable. Try closing your eyes to help you focus and concentrate on your breathing pattern. When you open your eyes, look around. Become aware of the little thoughts and inner feelings that your serenity time takes you to.

· During your serenity time, think happy thoughts. Accentuate the positive. Plan your dreams. Or just breathe. The point of serenity time is to escape from your day into your self for a few minutes.

· While you're at work, close your office door if you can and grab some quiet time.

TRY THIS SERENITY TIME TECHNIQUE

- Find a quiet place in your home or garden.
- Set a relaxing mood. You may wish to light scented candles or play soft, soothing music.
- Sit in a comfortable chair, take your shoes off, and place your feet flat on the floor.
- Close your eyes and begin to take long, deep breaths. Feel your breath moving into your abdomen.
- Allow your shoulders to relax.
- Inhale deeply for a count of four, hold the breath for a count of two, and then exhale slowly for another count of four.
- Use all five senses to feel where you want to take your mind. Imagine a favorite place, such as an ocean beach or a mountaintop. Feel the sun warming your skin and the gentle breeze blowing your hair, smell and taste the air, and hear the sounds of nature.
- Try this for two to three minutes and gradually work up to ten minutes or more.

- Take a serenity bath! Go ahead and schedule it in your planner if you have to, but start taking regular baths. From candlelit bubble baths to aromatherapy baths, nothing beats the sensation of warm water cleansing and calming your body and soul. According to *The New England Journal of Medicine*, soaking daily in a warm bath reduces blood sugar levels by 13 percent, slashes insulin needs by almost 20 percent, and can help women with diabetes lose 4 pounds of body fat in just three weeks. A surprising research study at New Orleans' Tulane University shows that soaking in warm water for as little as ten minutes is so effective at boosting blood and oxygen flow to the heart that it increases the heart's ability to pump blood by almost 20 percent. This benefits not only your heart, but the oxygen flow to your brain, your skin, and every other organ.

TRY THE FOLLOWING BATHS FOR YOUR SERENITY TIME

PAMPER-ME BATH:
Indulge your senses. Light a few candles in the bathroom, put on soft music, pour in a few drops of your favorite bath oil, and throw a few rose petals on top. Cover your closed eyes with cucumber slices or tea bags to draw out puffiness. Indulge!

BATH TO HELP YOU SLEEP AND RELAX MUSCLES:
Enhance your bath with tension-taming lavender oil. Mix 1 cup of Epsom salts (this soothes your muscles) with three drops of lavender oil in a warm bathtub. Toss in a few flower petals if you like. You will be sleepy-eyed within fifteen minutes!

CREAMY MILK BATH:

Pour ½ cup of milk under running bathwater. Wrap a sliced orange in cheesecloth, a coffee filter, or a thick paper towel, and squeeze it under the running water to release the orange oil. Add a few drops of vanilla extract and you're in soft, creamy heaven!

DETOX AND WEIGHT LOSS BATH:

Fill the tub half full with warm water and add 1 cup of baking soda. Do this for ten consecutive days, soaking for twenty minutes each day. This bath reduces toxins in your body, relieves stress, makes your skin feel baby smooth, and enhances weight loss. (Bath suggested by Marilu Henner in *The 30 Day Total Health Makeover*.)

PEPPERMINT POWER BATH:

Thanks to menthol, the main component in peppermint, a few drops of peppermint oil in your bath are sure to invigorate your senses and ease tired limbs.

FEEL-BETTER SALT BATH:

A scoop of mineral-rich bath salts will gently rinse away dull, flaky skin. These minerals can help alleviate minor aches and pains.

CHITCHAT

In researching the calming effects of serenity baths (OK, I admit I absolutely loved this assignment!) I have come to love my bath time and actually schedule it into my daily to-do list. As the mother of two young daughters, I decided to pass on this new tradition to my girls. Instead of their nightly cleansing bath, on occasion I allow them a special candlelit serenity bath, whereby we turn off the lights, light up a candle, and sip apple juice out of small cups from their tea set while they soak in a lavender-scented bath. Sometimes we even pick petals from the flower garden to throw in to make the event more festive! It's never too late or too early to begin healthy traditions!

—Lisa Lelas

The Key: Attaching This Step to Your Current Lifestyle

- Hang a positive affirmation on your dresser mirror as a reminder to take a few moments every morning as you awake to center yourself. Think about how you will keep your life in balance today. If you know that you will be having a hectic day ahead, think about how you can squeeze some relaxation time into your day.
- Establishing a particular time of day for your daily serenity time is the easiest way for you to continue with it on a regular basis.
- Make your serenity bath time a daily or weekly ritual. Sunday evenings, for example, can become "Mom's time" for an hour

or so. Dad can enjoy some special time out with the kids or rent a movie while you get the bathroom for a specific time period.

- Display a picture of a place you've always wanted to visit on the wall where you can see it from your bathtub or from your bed. This will help trigger your subconscious to take you away during your serenity time.

- Wake up twenty minutes earlier every day to enjoy a cup of calming herb tea and morning serenity time. Depending on what time it is, you might be able to enjoy a serenity sunrise to boot!

- If you find your own unique way to attach this step to your personal lifestyle, please share your ideas with us on our Web site: www.SimpleStepsProgram.com.

Sharing

Simple Steps Helped Peggy Get
Out of the Fast Lane and Relax

When Peggy remarried and moved to a new town, she felt a bit dis-connected. She wanted a more intimate bond with her new com-munity but seemed to find only superficial friendships. At the same time, she was juggling long hours at work and taking care of her home and family. It was exhausting.

Peggy remembers those days clearly. So much has happened since then. She had three goals at the time: get pregnant, lose weight, and slow down. It all seemed impossible before she joined the Simple Steps program. "I was running in seventeen different directions at the same time and not accomplishing anything. I was exhausted and wasn't feeling great about my life," she says.

Being on the road all day at her sales job kept her eating her meals in the car in between appointments. At home, she was mom to her eight-year-old son and her husband's ten- and twelve-year-old boys, all from their first marriages. What she wanted more than anything was a baby in this new marriage. But who had the time? Peggy was stressed at home and work. Everything seemed chaotic and disorganized.

Peggy lacked energy and she felt as though she was constantly out of breath. In fact, she believes that learning how to breathe correctly is one of the things she learned on the Simple Steps program that has become a healthy habit. When everything seemed to start spinning out of control, Peggy says, she learned to center herself, slow down, and take a breath.

Peggy found comfort in attending the Simple Steps meetings. She had an outlet to talk about her anxieties and her fear of not getting pregnant. She had been trying for quite a while without success and was now taking fertility pills. "I felt like I really could connect with these women, from the very beginning," she recalls. "There was just an openness there. Everyone was just up-front about what was going on in their lives. People talked about hurdles they got over, marital issues, ways they dealt with things. We just bonded. It was unique."

Step by step, Peggy felt herself taking charge of her life. "I never used to make my bed. I didn't see the sense in it. I didn't understand it was one of the many little things that were making me feel bad and disorganized. Now, making my bed is how I start my day. Every day. I feel so much better when I've done that one thing and I have a beautiful bed waiting for me in the evening."

As part of the first focus group for Simple Steps, Peggy was featured on *The Oprah Winfrey Show*, in a segment called "In the Spirit." In the piece, she explained how she found inner peace through her lifestyle makeover group. She was able to communicate more effectively with her husband, create new friendships, and simply feel better.

Then something truly wonderful happened. In week ten of the Simple Steps program, Peggy's wish came true. She was pregnant. "I was so excited," she remembers. "Maybe it was because Simple Steps helped me to relax and refocus—I can't say for sure, but what I do know is that I had a comfortable place to go where people would listen. I slowed down the pace of my life a little. I was feeling good, and then it happened."

Today, Peggy's little girl keeps her on her toes. "Some days I am still running, but I have learned to make priority lists. If it's not on my A-list of things that have to get done today, I move it to the next day's list and I don't panic. The important things in my life get done, and I'm making sure I have time to really stop and enjoy my family and my life."

Congratulations!

You've now mastered the following Simple Steps. Read them aloud as a positive affirmation. Make them a habit and keep them up as part of your new lifestyle.

I am drinking eight cups of water daily

I am walking twenty minutes a day

I am clearing out one drawer/cabinet/closet space every week

I am saving $2 a day (or 1 percent of my weekly salary)

I am keeping a daily food journal

I am squeezing in some isometrics every day

I am maintaining an efficient laundry system

I am following a daily to-do list

I am taking a multivitamin every day

I am aware of my posture and breathing

I am keeping a clear desktop

I am cleansing and moisturizing daily

I am replacing bad fats with good fats

I am dancing to at least one song every day

I am maintaining a clean and healthy refrigerator and pantry

I am cleaning and flossing my teeth twice daily

I am cutting back on caffeine

I am discovering the benefits of yoga

I am maintaining a system to avoid mail piles

I am finding daily serenity time

WEEK SIX

The Tulip

Simple grace. Soft and feminine.
An enchanting spirit.

Trading Carbs

Find Healthy Alternatives to Processed Carbohydrates

Why Do We Need to Be Careful About What Kind of Carbohydrates We Eat?

- Only 3 percent of all Americans meet at least four of the five federal Food Guide Pyramid recommendations for the intake of grains, fruits, and vegetables, according to the U.S. Department of Health and Human Services. Are you one of them?
- We need to trade our bagged and boxed foods for whole grains, fruits, and vegetables because it is healthier, we will look and feel better, and we will enjoy increased energy.
- We need at least 25 grams of dietary fiber a day, according to the U.S. Food and Drug Administration. Fifty-five percent of our total calories should be from natural complex carbohydrates such as whole grains, vegetables, fruit, and legumes. It is easy to get our 25 grams of dietary fiber into our day by making better choices.
- There is a big difference between natural carbohydrates, found in whole grains, such as brown rice and whole wheat, and the carbohydrates found in enriched (also known as "refined") grains. Natural carbohydrates offer more fiber, vitamins, and

minerals. Enriched foods are processed, which means nutrients are added, but often so are unwanted ingredients. Watch
out for sodium, sugar, partially hydrogenated oils, nitrites,
MSG, and sulfur.

· Unrefined carbohydrates are absorbed into our bloodstream
slowly and hence provide a steady energy level. Refined carbs
and sugars go directly into our bloodstream, causing fast sugar
highs of energy followed by deep lows, which often lead to
overeating.

· Obesity and type 2 diabetes are becoming epidemic in American society due largely to consumption of sugar and refined
or processed food products, according to Health Education
Alliance for Life and Longevity, www.heall.com. Americans
eat the equivalent of 20 teaspoons of sugar a day, reports the
federal *Continuing Survey of Food Intakes by Individuals*, cited
in an article from the U.S. Food and Drug Administration,
November–December 1999.

· By replacing bad carbohydrates with good, and thereby taking
in more fiber, we are helping to prevent constipation, hemorrhoids, and bacterial infections by keeping the contents of the
intestine moist and flushed out.

· Fiber can help reduce blood cholesterol and blood sugars. It
also may benefit conditions and diseases like diabetes, bowel
irregularity (constipation or diarrhea), macular degeneration,
and hiatal hernia.

· *Soluble fiber* dissolves in water. It helps to reduce blood cholesterol and blood sugars. Soluble fiber foods include barley,
fruits (especially apples, strawberries, oranges, bananas, nec-
tarines, and pears), legumes, oats, oat bran, rye, seeds, and
vegetables (especially carrots, corn, cauliflower, and sweet
potatoes).

· *Insoluble fiber* does not dissolve in water as quickly. It helps maintain regularity, regulates bowel movements, helps food move quickly through the small intestine, and reduces the risk of colon cancer, hemorrhoids, and appendicitis. Insoluble fiber foods include brown rice, fruits, legumes, seeds, wheat bran, whole grains, and vegetables (especially potatoes with skin, parsnips, green beans, and broccoli).

- Fiber can help in weight control. We feel full when we eat fiber-rich foods because they absorb water and swell.
- Food products high in refined carbohydrates and low in vitamins are called "empty calories," otherwise known as junk food. They only add pounds. It is important to trade your empty calories for food rich in natural carbohydrates.

CHITCHAT

I remember a simple science experiment I did back in the fourth grade. Our teacher gave us each a saltine cracker to place in our mouth. We had to let it dissolve on our tongue without chewing it. After a few minutes passed, I remember being amazed as my salty cracker began to taste sweet. The carbohydrates were breaking down and turning into sugar right before my eyes . . . or should I say in my mouth! We have been giving this assignment to our Simple Steps groups to try at home, and the women who try it say they can now see that white flour really does instantly become sugar! —Lisa Lelas

How to Trade Carbs

- If you're an oatmeal lover, try trading your rolled oats for steel-cut oats because they are still in the raw state with the hull intact.
- Add wheat germ or ground flaxseed to your cereal for extra nutrition and extra flavor.
- Trade your high-sugar cereal for a cereal low in sugar (under 3 grams per serving) and high in fiber (over 4 grams per serving). Read your labels.
- If you like muffins or Danish for breakfast, trade them in for a fresh fruit salad or a whole wheat bagel.
- Drink herbal tea instead of drinking a can of soda, which can have approximately 8 teaspoons of sugar in it.
- Trade in your sugared and sulfured dried fruits for the natural dried fruits without the additives.
- Instead of having a pasta dish with a cheese sauce, opt for a whole wheat or artichoke pasta dish with a seafood marinara sauce. You can also serve this marinara on top of brown rice.
- Discover legumes! Throw them together with a serving of brown rice and vegetables and you will have a great meal that tastes great and is full of fiber and natural carbohydrates.
- Instead of having cake or ice cream for dessert, have a handful of fruit.
- Use natural sugars such as honey, blackstrap molasses, and maple syrup in place of refined sugar. Although they are considered a simple sugar, they have nutrients in them. Use these sparingly; they are high in calories. Consider adding foods such as dates, raisins, or other sweet fruits when baking, so you can cut back on sugar.

- Buy natural whole products such as legumes, fruits, and vegetables, instead of buying these products canned. During the canning process, many additives are included to hinder spoiling, and the heating process tends to cook out some natural vitamins and minerals. If you can't buy these products fresh, second best is frozen. Most food products are flash frozen while they are in a fresh state, so nutrients freeze with the product.

The Key: Attaching This Step to Your Current Lifestyle

- Check your food journal to make sure you're eating at least six servings of whole grain products; two fruits, and at least four vegetables each day. Eating your recommended daily amounts may help curb your cravings for junk food.
- While cleaning out your pantry, pack up all of your refined/processed products and give them to your local food shelter. Replace these food products with natural and whole grain products.
- In the grocery store, when you reach for your next purchase of bread, pasta, or rice, be sure to buy the whole grain product: whole grain bread, whole wheat pasta, and brown rice.
- When you are looking for a snack, instead of grabbing a bag of processed chips, grab a mouthwatering piece of fruit (fresh, not canned) or a handful of cut-up vegetables. Vegetables not only have a lot of fiber, but they also have an abundance of vitamins and minerals to satisfy your dietary needs.
- Keep a container of fresh vegetables in your refrigerator so when you need something to grab fast, you won't have an excuse to grab a bag of chips.

- Get your family involved. It's easier to trade carbs when your family is behind you. If you shouldn't have it, more than likely your family shouldn't.
- If you find your own unique way to attach this step to your personal lifestyle, please share your ideas with us on our Web site: www.SimpleStepsProgram.com.

Crunches

Do a Few Minutes of Crunches Every Day

Why Should We Do Crunches?

- Crunches help develop strong abdominal muscles, which can help us look slimmer and healthier by getting those flabby bellies trim. Belly bulges are amplified by poor posture and weak abs.
- Our abdominal muscles are the wide, flat muscles that run from our breastbone to the front of our pelvis. Strong abdominal muscles will help us maintain a healthy back, which will improve our posture and can reduce back pain and the risk of back injury.
- Crunches can make other physical activities easier. In martial arts, strong abs are necessary because we are constantly rotating our body. In running, strong abs help keep your hips square so that our leg action is forward and back.
- No matter how much we diet and exercise, our abdominal muscles need direct attention to be strengthened and toned.

How to Do Crunches

- Lie flat on your back on a mat, a towel, or a carpeted floor.
- Bend your knees and put your feet flat on the floor.
- Place your hands behind your head or across your chest and keep your eyes focused on the ceiling. Take in a deep breath.
- As you exhale, raise your upper body off the floor by squeezing your abdominal muscles. Do not lift with your neck and head; make sure these remain loose and relaxed. You are raising your shoulders off the floor with your abdominal muscles; you are not coming up to a full sit-up.
- Proper breathing is essential. As you crunch up, exhale. Try to imagine you are squeezing all of the air out of your midsection, as if you were deflating a balloon. Inhale as you slowly lower yourself back down.
- Repeat three sets of eight crunches.
- As you progress, try picking your feet up off the floor by either tucking your knees into your chest or bringing your feet straight up (eventually you will be able to hold your legs at a 45-degree angle from the floor). The flatter your back is against the floor, the harder the workout will be for your abs.
- While you're crunching, try doing the bicycle. Keeping your feet off the floor and your hands by your ears, move one knee in toward your chest as you bring your opposite elbow as close as you can get to that knee, with your shoulders raised off the floor and your abs tight. Slowly bring that leg and elbow down to the starting position—feet still off the floor—and rotate to the other side. This exercise will work your back and oblique muscles (the muscles that cover your ribs and sides).
- Another variation is the stand-up crunch. Stand with your feet and legs in a comfortable position, cross your arms in front of

your chest (hands to elbows), and tilt your pelvic muscles out so that your back is flat. Slowly turn from side to side with your abdominal muscles clenched tight. Turn only as far as your muscles will let you without strain. Slowly move back to face the front and repeat with the other side. Start with two sets of eight repetitions and work up to three sets of twelve repetitions.

The Key: Attaching This Step to Your Current Lifestyle

- Begin your day by doing your crunches right after you get out of bed.
- While the water for your shower is getting warm or while you wait for your morning cup of tea to brew, get on the floor and do one set of eight crunches.
- Practice stand-up crunches while taking your shower.
- Do your crunches during commercial breaks while watching TV.
- Do crunches before or after your daily walk.
- Hang an outfit or a bikini you'd love to look good in where you can see it when you open your closet door, to remind you to do those crunches.
- Place a magazine picture of a model with sculpted abs on the refrigerator or bathroom mirror.
- When watching your evening news program, make it a point to do your crunches during the weather report.
- You might have a beautiful six-pack of abdominal muscles, but you will never see them under too much fat. Keep walking and stay on a healthy diet to show off your hard work.
- If you find your own unique way to attach this step to your personal lifestyle, please share your ideas with us on our Web site: www.SimpleStepsProgram.com.

A Clean Car

Clean Out Your Car

Why Should We Clean Out Our Car?

- Our automobile is one of the spaces outside of our home where we spend a great deal of time. In essence, it is an extension of our home and should be housecleaned regularly and maintained daily. We feel better when our car is clean and orderly just like our home.

- A clean car gives us a sense of control and power. We feel in charge and ready to face the world, instead of being lost and buried in clutter.

- The condition of our car is a direct reflection of *us*. Like it or not, the outside world sometimes judges us by the surroundings they see us in.

- A clean car can improve our mood. A cluttered, messy car filled with disheveled papers and trash, misplaced mail, receipts, and empty water bottles can cause stress and frustration.

- A clean car means we know where things are the moment we may need them. We can find things such as our insurance card, a map, or change for the toll.

- A thoroughly cleaned car is a wise investment. Keeping our car clean can up its resale value and remove those end-of-lease excess-wear-and-tear charges. That should get you motivated.

- A clean car smells better than a dirty car.

WEIGHT LOSS TIP

In a totally nonscientific survey, we found through our Simple Steps group participants that women actually ate less when their cars were clean! When their cars were scrubbed showroom clean inside and out, they no longer wanted to snack while driving in the car or stop at fast-food drive-through restaurants for fear of crumbs and litter. *Many admitted they actually craved less food in general as they gained this piece of control in their lives. Something to think about!*

How to Clean Your Car

- First, gather your supplies: a vacuum cleaner or handheld vacuum, a glass cleaner, a soft cloth or chamois, an oil-based soap for leather seats, a bucket filled with water and a few drops of dish-washing liquid or a specific car cleaner such as Turtle Wax, a hose with a power nozzle, a scrub sponge, clean dry towels, and two brown paper trash bags.
- Start by organizing and discarding any useless clutter or garbage. Be thorough with two brown grocery bags in hand, one for saving items to be put away elsewhere, and the other for trash. Then get to work cleaning this home away from home!
- Take out all floor mats and shake them out.

CHATTER TIME

Melissa, a mother of three, finally figured out a solution for keeping the floor of her car clean. Once a year she purchases small carpet squares from her local dollar store (sometimes you can find free scrap samples from rug dealers) and uses them over her manufacturer's rug mats. At the end of a messy fall-winter season (snow, mud, salt), she simply discards the squares and purchases new ones.

· Using a dustcloth, wipe the dash and all plastic or vinyl surfaces. Then wipe them down with a sponge damp with dishwashing soap and water (squeeze the sponge out).

· If you have a leather interior, use oil-based soap cleaner to gently wipe down the seats.

· Vacuum the interior of the car, including seats, carpeting, and the trunk.

· When you are cleaning the exterior of your car, always hose off the loose dirt first. Then, with sponge in hand, suds up one section of the car at a time and rinse off. Use a separate sponge for really grimy areas such as the wheels.

· Using your soft cloth, mop up all dampness to dry it before water spots appear.

· Wash the car windows inside and out with a glass cleaner and a soft, dry towel.

· When taking your car to a professional car wash, consider a soft-cloth wash or a touchless car wash if you are worried about scratching.

· Suggested items to keep inside your automobile: your vehicle's registration and your insurance cards, a tire pressure gauge, a flashlight, a list of emergency telephone numbers, a first aid kit, a pen, a road map, change for tolls, a multipurpose tool (like the Swiss Army AutoTool), and a cellular telephone with charger and hands-free talk kit.

- Other items to consider carrying: moist towelettes, sunglasses, nonperishable food items (such as PowerBars and packaged trail mixes), bottled water, a blanket, an umbrella, and, if you live in colder, northern climates, an ice scraper, extra gloves, and a small shovel.
- If you have the room, a bin under the backseat is a great organizer for kid's snacks, wipes, and Band-Aids.
- If you have very young kids, keep an extra diaper bag in the car stocked with diapers, wipes, a blanket, and car toys.
- Organizational pouches, available for hanging on the back of front seats, are great for creating an activity zone for children—by storing books and car games—or for storing road maps and tissues.
- Get a handy CD or audiotape case that can fit under the passenger seat.
- Hang a small sachet of lavender and rosemary somewhere on your dash. The scent not only is relaxing but helps keep you focused while driving.
- Put baking soda or potpourri into the ashtray to make the interior smell fresh.
- In the trunk of your car keep emergency tools, a spare tire, spare fuses, jumper cables, a blanket, and bungee cords for securing any hard-to-carry items, such as furniture.
- Keep a garbage bag inside your car for daily upkeep.
- Never let anyone smoke in your car. That smell will lower the value of the car.

The Key: **Attaching This Step to Your Current Lifestyle**

- If an organizational system is in place in your car, you will use it without a second thought. For example, if you use your car for your job or run many errands throughout the day, a shallow basket in the passenger seat next to you is great for holding your purse, letters to mail, a map that you're using, etc.
- For families with children, assign a small paper gift bag to each child, to be folded and kept neatly by their seat. When exiting the car, all children are to throw their stuff into their gift bag and carry it *out* of the car. This might include books, sip cups, empty snack bags, or a banana peel.
- Always remove clutter (empty coffee cups, gum wrappers, etc.) every time you leave your car.
- Keep reminding yourself that it's simple to maintain a car's cleanliness once you've cleared everything out.
- Set up a regular cleaning day for your car. Running by the car wash on Mondays, on your way to the market, or to your son's soccer game is a good routine to establish.
- If you find your own unique way to attach this step to your personal lifestyle please share your ideas with us on our Web site: www.SimpleStepsProgram.com.

Dressing Smart

Update Your Look
and Your Closet

Why Should We Dress Smart and Update Our Closet?

- Dressing smart means paying attention to the clothes we wear every day, making sure they are clean and crisp, fit properly, suit our needs, and reflect our own personal style.
- The clothes we choose to wear speak volumes about us—our values, our tastes, and our self-image. What do we want our outfit to *say*?
- An up-to-date image may help us feel more put together and attractive.
- We can look slimmer when we wear the proper attire, since our clothes will fit better and hang properly on our frame.
- We wear 20 percent of our clothing 80 percent of the time, according to Mary Lou Andre, wardrobe consultant, speaker, author, and founder and president of Organization By Design in Needham, Massachusetts. This means that 80 percent of our clothing is just cluttering our closet.
- An updated closet means having a clean and organized space that allows you to view your entire wardrobe (or at least to view

your summer wardrobe in the spring and summer, and your
winter wardrobe in fall and winter).
- An organized closet saves us time by allowing us to find what
we're looking for when we need it.
- A well-dressed woman reflects confidence and grace. We can
achieve a polished look by updating our wardrobe.
- We simply feel better about ourselves when our closet is up-to-
date and we dress smart.

How to Dress Smart

- When purchasing clothes, concentrate on quality rather than
quantity. Better clothes last longer and look better in the long
run. Quality clothing drapes better and retains shape after
being washed. You're better off with one good outfit that you
love and fits you well than three inexpensive ones that are not
comfortable and don't fit well.
- Buy your basics first. Purchase quality slacks, skirts, and jack-
ets in black, navy blue, or tan. Basic items in neutral colors are
more versatile than trendy clothing, which goes out of style.
- Once you have the basics, add sweaters, blouses, and accessories.
- Accessories can be used to add color to an outfit. Pull together
an outfit using matching shoes, scarf, and jewelry.
- Move beyond black, especially in summer and spring, but use
bright colors sparingly. Soft, quiet colors blend with more outfits.
- Simplicity is elegant and timeless. Choose clothes that are
comfortable and easy to wear.
- Choose smooth fabrics, because they layer well when the
weather starts to cool.

- Avoid wearing the right things the wrong way. For instance, you should be able to insert two fingers into the waistband of pants or a skirt for a comfortable fit. Wearing items that are too small or too tight can make you appear heavier than you really are.
- Always check labels and be sure your purchases are machine washable to simplify your life. You will make fewer trips to the dry cleaner and spend less time ironing.
- Clothing experts recommend shopping no more than twice a year for clothes, once in the fall and once in the spring. This eliminates impulse shopping and can save you money.
- Review your wardrobe and decide what you need for the season you are shopping for. Perhaps you want new tops in the hottest seasonal colors, or maybe you need to replace your favorite pair of black slacks. Perhaps a new sweater will add that special something to last year's basic outfit. Just be sure you know what you are looking for before you go to the store.
- Browse, browse, and browse. Look through fashion magazines and window-shop at clothing stores. Don't buy until you really know what you want.
- When you shop for nice clothes, dress up. Wear the undergarments you plan to wear with the new outfit so you will be able to judge your look when you try on items in the dressing room.
- Try on even those items that you would never think to buy. You might be surprised how they make you look and feel.
- A sagging bust can add 10 pounds and up to ten years to your look. Look for a bra that lifts your bust. Most women's bra size changes during their life. Take the following steps to determine your appropriate bra size:
  - Determine your number size by measuring around your chest, under your bustline. Round off to the closest inch. If the number is even, add 4 inches; if it is odd, add 5.

- To determine your cup size, measure the fullest part of your bust and round off to the closest inch. Subtract the number size (calculated in step one) from this measurement. If you get 0 to ½, you are an AA cup; 1, A cup; 2, B cup; 3, C cup; 4, D cup; and 5, DD or E cup.

- Here's an example: If the measurement around your chest is 32½, round it off to 33. Since this is an odd number, add 5 inches to equal 38. If the measurement around the fullest part of your breast is 40½, round it off to 41. Then subtract 38, your number size, from 41. This means your bra size is 38 C.

How to Update Your Closet

- Stop, organize, and gain control. Investing time to review your wardrobe now will save you time each day standing in front of your closet wondering what to wear.
- Take time to plan out closet organization before you begin.
- If your closet is tall enough, hang two rods: one around 7 feet high for dresses and pants, and another at 3½ feet high for skirts, blouses, and shorter items.
- Empty everything from your closet. Place each clothing item into one of four piles on the floor: clothes to be rehung or re-folded, clothes to go to dry cleaner/tailor, clothes to be given to charity or friends, and clothes to be discarded.
- Place charity donations in a black plastic bag and put it in your car so you'll be sure to drop it off. If you keep these items in your room, they might creep back into your closet.
- If you have not worn something in two years and forgot you even had it, give it away. If it's stained, no longer fits, or is beyond repair, throw it away.
- When replacing clothing items, remember, every single item in

your closet should be stored in plain sight. If you don't see it, you won't wear it. So don't overcrowd your closet with too many new things.

- Some women like to arrange their clothing according to what they use during the week versus the weekend.

- Others like to categorize their clothes by grouping like items together (all skirts in one section, blouses in another, etc.) or by sorting items according to color, length, or style.

- Others like to put together outfits that match so they can grab a whole ensemble and go!

- Sort through your accessories and get rid of items you no longer use.

- If you have certain accessories you always wear with a particular outfit, store them with the outfit by attaching a plastic sandwich bag to the hanger.

- Organize shoes in your closet. If you keep your shoes in boxes, label the box or take a picture of the shoes and tape it to the outside of the box. Store boots and shoes with their tops facing each other, heel to toe, to save space.

- Place a favorite soap in a mesh bag and hang it in your closet for a clean fresh smell. Lavender scent will discourage moths and keep stored items smelling nice.

The Key: Attaching This Step to Your Current Lifestyle

- Mark your calendar for two weekends during the year to shop for new clothes. The week before each trip, refresh the organization of your closet and make a list of new things you need.

- Hang a write-on board in your closet to make notes of clothing in need of repair or other items you need to add to your wardrobe. If you see items you would like to buy before your biannual shopping trip, cut out pictures or make a list so you don't forget to look for them when you shop.

- Remove one old garment from your closet for every new item you add.
- Expand your wardrobe by wearing all the clothes in your closet.
- Get into the habit of hanging your clothes up or putting them in the hamper as soon as you change.
- Plan ahead. Choose your clothes the night before. Think about where your day might take you. Dress according to your plans.
- Your wardrobe should make *your* fashion statement. Shop alone so others won't influence the statement you're trying to make or encourage you to buy things you can't afford.
- If you find your own unique way to attach this step to your personal lifestyle, please share your ideas with us on our Web site: www.SimpleStepsProgram.com.

Sharing

Simple Steps Turned This
Cluttered Pack Rat into
"Little Miss Suzy Homemaker"!

When Suzy began the Simple Steps program, she felt as though she had found a piece of herself that had been missing since childhood.

From the time she was five years old, Suzy was already being trained to be a physician. "I was an academic commando," she remembers. "After I grew up and actually became a doctor, my life became extremely organized. When my three children were in diapers, I was working fifty hours a week. I had someone for day care. I had someone take care of the house. I left at seven in the morning, came home at seven at night, read them a story, and tucked them into bed."

Suzy says at some point she realized this was not how she wanted to live. She wanted to stay home with her children. "That wouldn't necessarily be the right choice for everyone, but I knew it was the right choice for me. Staying home and dealing with all the emotional ups and downs of your kids' day and taking care of a household, in my opinion, is definitely more difficult than going to work, but I ultimately felt I couldn't work and raise my children the way I wanted to."

The problem was Suzy didn't know a lot about running a household. "I love to cook," she explains. "I started making fancy meals every night, but nobody ever showed me how to fold laundry, clean a floor, or organize closets. You've seen the cartoons where you open a closet door and everything falls out on your head. At first I figured, oh well, I just don't do that very well. It doesn't matter. I'm a nice person; people like me. But after a while, I knew my husband was unhappy coming home to a messy house. He asked if I wanted to go back to work so we could hire someone to keep our house in order." Suzy finally realized her system of having *no* systems was simply not working.

When Suzy heard about the Simple Steps program, she was ready. She wanted to lose some weight, get some personal motivation back, and learn how to organize her home. "I just started following the program week by week and instantly started feeling better. One of the things that ties people like me up is the idea that if you can't make it perfect right away, why bother? I learned that it doesn't have to be perfect today. Each little change will have its own impact. Once you have a space organized, it doesn't take much to come back a week or two later and straighten it up. You aren't starting over again."

As Suzy's home became more organized, she started dropping weight. "Once again, I didn't do anything radical. I just learned to think about eating healthier and drinking water, and I started exercising." Suzy started with the walking assignment and got such great results, she took it to a higher level. Now she's working out at a gym, lifting weights and sometimes working with a trainer. She's lost 25 pounds.

Suzy claims her husband thinks Simple Steps is a miracle. "It's really changed the way he feels about coming home. And it's certainly changed the way I feel about myself. I love coming home to a house where the counters are clean and I can start cooking without having to clear away a pile of junk mail. We all have to make choices in our lives. I don't think we can necessarily have it all at the same time. Right now, I know I am living the best life I can."

Congratulations!

You've now mastered the following Simple Steps. Read them aloud
as a positive affirmation. Make them a habit and keep them up as
part of your new lifestyle.

I am drinking eight cups of water daily

I am walking twenty minutes a day

I am clearing out one drawer/cabinet/closet space every week

I am saving $2 a day (or 1 percent of my weekly salary)

I am keeping a daily food journal

I am squeezing in some isometrics every day

I am maintaining an efficient laundry system

I am following a daily to-do list

I am taking a multivitamin every day

I am aware of my posture and breathing

I am keeping a clear desktop

I am cleansing and moisturizing daily

I am replacing bad fats with good fats

I am dancing to at least one song every day

I am maintaining a clean and healthy refrigerator and pantry

I am cleaning and flossing my teeth twice daily

I am cutting back on caffeine
I am discovering the benefits of yoga
I am maintaining a system to avoid mail piles
I am finding daily serenity time
I am replacing processed foods with whole grains
I am doing a few minutes of crunches every day
I am maintaining a clean car
I am dressing smart and keeping my closet organized

The
Morning
Glory

Forever faithful.
A sunrise spectacular.

Honoring Food

Eat Less by Slowing Down and Savoring Every Bite

Why Is It Important to Honor Food?

- Food keeps us alive. We must eat to live, but we shouldn't live to eat. Slowing down and honoring our food during meals helps us remember these truths.
- It takes our stomachs approximately twenty minutes to signal our brain that it is full. The faster we eat, the *more* we eat. Eating too fast significantly increases our chance of overeating.
- The first bite always tastes the best. Once we swallow, we no longer taste food. So chew carefully and thoroughly and savor your food.
- Meals should be a pleasurable experience. Does your whole family sit down? Why rush? Slow down and make the pleasurable experience last.
- If we need to unbutton our pants after a meal, we definitely ate too much and it was probably because we ate too fast.
- Consuming food too fast increases the chance of experiencing heartburn or gastric reflux.
- The longer we chew food, the better our digestion. Eating more

slowly will increase the saliva mixing with food in our mouth to begin the digestive process.

· Being a member of the clean-plate club can make a huge difference in our waistlines, according to a recent survey done by the American Institute for Cancer Research. The survey found 67 percent of Americans eat everything on their plate—even if they are full. And remember, 61 percent of adult Americans are overweight.

· Not eating one-quarter of the food on your plate will reduce both fat and calories in your diet. Especially when you go to restaurants, remember that you don't have to eat it just because it's there!

How to Slow Down, Eat Less, and Honor Food

· Before you start eating, pause to be grateful for the food on your plate and treat it with respect.

· Make a fist with your right hand and hold it up in front of you. Take your left hand and wrap your fingers around your right wrist. The fist you are holding up (only from the wrist up) is approximately the same size as your stomach. Keep this in mind when deciding how much to eat at each meal. All portions should be able to fit into the mold of your fist.

· Were you taught to clean your plate at every meal? If you were, we ask that you now consider giving up your membership in the clean-plate club. Remember you can always save food for later. Leftovers from dinner often make a great lunch for tomorrow.

· Begin your meal with a hot bowl of soup. Soup will curb your appetite as well as force you to slow down because of its temperature. A study conducted by Baylor College of Medicine in

Houston found that those who consumed a hot bowl of soup before meals ate less, lost more weight, and kept it off longer.

- Avoid serving dinner family style. Having extra food on the table will only entice you to have seconds. Leave the food on the stove and serve everyone's portions on their plates. Better yet, also put away any leftovers before sitting down to eat.
- Taste a small amount of each type of food on your plate and rate each from favorite to least favorite. Eat the food you like best first, saving your least favorite for last. It's easier to leave something on your plate that has less appeal to your taste buds.
- When you eat, take smaller bites and savor each mouthful. When you feel satisfied, stop eating. Never eat until you are full.
- Stop midmeal and talk with your family for fifteen minutes. Many times you will not go back to your meal, because after this break, it's easier to realize you feel satisfied by what you have already eaten.
- Don't skip meals, or your hunger will push you to eat too fast.
- Never eat anything standing up to prevent mindless eating. Keep this in mind when cooking.
- Get into the habit of chewing food thoroughly.
- When eating at a restaurant, ask for a leftovers bag. Save one-half of your meal for tomorrow's lunch.
- Next time you think about taking another serving, hold up your fist and ask yourself, "Will another serving fit comfortably into the mold of my hand?"
- Don't eat anything that is not *delicious* to you.

CHATTER TIME

Rita found her own unique way to change her eating habits and shared the following tip with the group. She would set the clock timer in her kitchen for twenty minutes at the beginning of each meal. Her goal was to have some food left on her plate when the buzzer sounded. At first, the twenty-minute timer seemed incredibly slow, and Rita had a hard time making meals last, but her determination paid off. After about two weeks, she was happy to report to the class that it was now a breeze to make meals last twenty minutes. Rita was also happy to report that because she ate more slowly, she was satisfied with less food and ate less. Now it has become a daily habit for her to leave food on her plate.

The Key: Attaching This Step to Your Current Lifestyle

- Make it a habit to never eat anything out of the bag or box it comes in. Pour one serving into a bowl or on a plate. If you eat straight from the bag or box, it's likely you will eat more than one serving.
- Turn off the television and radio during meals. Don't allow yourself to be distracted from your food or you might eat unconsciously. Quiet conversations with friends or family, or simple contemplation are the best accompaniments to your meals.
- Turn on the lights during meals to raise your attention level and to focus on your food.

- When eating at home, use a salad plate rather than a dinner plate.
- Slow down your eating by using the opposite hand of the one you usually eat with. If you are right-handed, eat meals with the fork in your left hand. This will force you to slow down.
- Put your fork down between bites to further slow yourself down.
- Challenge yourself to leave some food on the plate at every meal.
- Keep sugarless gum or mints on hand. Chew gum or eat a mint as soon as you feel satisfied. It will wash the taste of food from your mouth and make after-dinner picking less appealing.
- Brush and floss your teeth immediately after each meal. You will have a brighter smile and be less likely to nibble after dinner.
- Make it a habit to tighten your belt before a big meal. You will eat less.
- When you know you will be tempted to overeat at a social event, wear fitted rather than loose clothing; you will have a constant reminder around your middle not to overeat.
- If you find your own unique way to attach this step to your personal lifestyle, please share your ideas with us on our Web site: www.SimpleStepsProgram.com.

Stretching

Greet Every Day with a Morning Stretch

Why Do We Need to Stretch?

- Stretching loosens stiff muscles, reducing tension and sore-ness and giving us greater flexibility.
- Stretching will increase our mobility as well as increase our total body relaxation.
- We can help prevent loss in flexibility as we get older if we stretch daily.
- When we exercise, our muscles plump up or contract, so we have to restretch our muscles to avoid becoming tight.
- Morning stretching gets our blood pumping and shakes off our sleepiness.
- We will feel good after our morning stretch, ready to take on the day ahead.

How to Stretch Every Morning

- Stretching can be done by people of all ages and fitness levels.
- If you are older, or haven't stretched in a while, you will proba-

bly need to be patient in getting the flexibility you want. Practice each day consistently and you'll be delighted to discover how quickly you improve.

- This simple daily morning stretch should be in addition to the yoga you're doing once a week.

- Hold stretches for a slow count of five and remember not to bounce.

- Breathe. Breathing helps relax your body and increase blood flow. Exhale as your muscles are stretching. While contracting your muscles, inhale slowly through your nose, expanding your abdomen, holding your breath for a moment. Exhale slowly, preferably through your nose. There should be no force of breath. If you are exhaling from your mouth, make an *ahhh* sound to be sure your breath is controlled.

- Do not stretch if you feel pain. You may feel a bit of discomfort at first, but stretch only at a level that feels comfortable to you.

- Be a copycat. Watch your cat, dog, or baby as he or she awakens with the natural instinct to stretch. We recommend starting your stretch routine when you first wake up in the morning, just like they do.

- Upon awakening, before your shower, stretch out for the day. Rotate your joints clockwise, then counterclockwise, including your shoulders, wrists, ankles, and elbows. Bend your arms and legs; bend at the knees and at the waist. Wake up your fingers and toes by clasping them open and closed a few times.

- While lying on your back with your toes pointed and your hands over your head, stretch your fingers as far as they can reach while your toes are pointing as far as they can go. Rotate sides, stretching left and then right. Hold each stretch for a few seconds each. If you don't have room on your bed, stretch on the floor.

- Lying on your back, bring one knee up to your chest and hug it with your arms. Repeat with other knee. Bring both knees into your chest and hug them for a nice back stretch.

- Another easy morning stretch is to bend side to side, which is good for your waistline. While standing with knees soft and feet shoulders' width apart, rest a broomstick on your shoulders behind your neck with both hands clasping it from behind. Gently bend sideways, tipping the broomstick down. Come back up and repeat other side. Try three reps of eight. You can also do this with a bath towel. Holding the towel above your head with your arms straight up, bend side to side. Or try bending sideways with your hands on your hips.

CHATTER TIME

We laughed until we cried when we pictured one full-figured participant (over age 65) as she explained her morning stretch routine. She shared with the group that before she dressed in the morning, she would go into her closet (so she wouldn't wake her husband) and use her bra as an exercise band. With her bra stretched high above her head, she bent side to side. As her flexibility increased, one morning she reached so far to one side that she knocked over a closet shelf. When her husband opened the closet door, he found her buried under a mound of winter sweaters and pocketbooks!

- Reach for your toes. Either sit on the floor or stand with your legs shoulder width apart (or wider), knees slightly bent. Gently reach for your knee or ankle (as far down your leg as you can go) with your opposite hand. Hold for a few seconds and repeat with the other side.

- Before and after your morning walk, stretch out your calf and thigh muscles by standing on a step with your heels hanging off the back of the step—slowly lower one heel at a time while you keep your toes on the step.

The Key: Attaching This Step to Your Current Lifestyle

- Every morning upon awakening, before you place your feet on the ground, stretch!
- Each morning try to reach the top of a window (or higher), stretching on your tiptoes as high as you can reach. Every morning try to reach a higher level on the wall.
- After brushing your teeth, while rinsing your mouth, do a set of waist twists.
- Stretch everywhere; be creative. On an airplane, during long flights, rotate your shoulders and ankles.
- While sitting at your desk, bend over and touch your toes.
- While standing in a long line, slowly rotate your head side to side.
- While waiting for an elevator, alternate stretching your upper arms across your chest while supporting your elbow with your opposite hand.
- While sitting and watching television, lift your legs one at a time, flexing and pointing your toes.
- Have your family join you for morning stretching before breakfast. This can be a fun family fitness ritual to do every morning.
- If you find your own unique way to attach this step to your personal lifestyle, please share your ideas with us on our Web site: www.SimpleStepsProgram.com.

Organizing Photos

Organize Your Photographs

Why Should We Organize Our Photos?

- Having disorganized photographs that are scattered around without labels or dates is one of the biggest and most common household clutter problems.
- Getting photos organized and displayed properly gives us a sense of control.
- Neatly displayed and updated photos release guilt. We have found this to be a common burden among women, especially mothers of teenagers who still feel a tug at their heartstrings for not having completed their children's baby books.
- Having organized photos keeps us connected to our loved ones, which can be especially important if they live far away or have passed on.
- Neatly matted and framed photographs, whether current or heirloom, warm our home and create a unique decor for every room.
- Organized photos give us freedom to find our precious memories quickly when we desire to share them with someone. For instance, at the dinner party when you and your guests begin to

reminisce about that trip to Paris you took together five years ago, you are able to quickly retrieve that travel album for sharing during dessert.

- Organized photographs are like artwork that gives us joy. We can see our memories come to life through the magic of time frozen onto 4-by-6-inch canvases.

How to Organize Your Photos

GETTING STARTED

- Visiting a photo supply or craft store is a good first step when beginning your photo-organizing journey. A few helpful purchases can go a long way toward simplifying the process. Invest in several photo storage boxes. These are better than shoe boxes because they are acid free and designed to protect photographs. Monthly divider cards are included in most. Purchase a few acid-free pens or markers for labeling the backs of photos, and a few acid-free glue sticks for securing photos in albums or journals. You may also want to pick up a few inexpensive, easy-to-use photo albums. If you have an overwhelming number of photos to organize, consider buying albums by the case. They are cheaper by the dozen. Look for the word *archival* on the packaging of photograph storage supplies. *Archival* means that the product will protect photos for one hundred years or more.
- Create a photo-organizing work zone in your home, preferably in a location that will allow you to leave your photos and supplies out and intact between work sessions. Depending on how many photographs you have, this step may need more than one week. Plan to give it at least one hour each week until you're done.
- Begin by gathering all the loose photographs in your home.

Depending upon how many photos you have, this may require a big box or bin.

- Now you are ready to begin sorting. Start from your most recent photographs and work back in time toward the old photos. Categorize them by date, even if you have to guess the approximate date or year. It is helpful to have labeled boxes for each year as a sorting tool. Then sort each box individually into season, month, or event.

- Next, file each group of photos from a particular season, month, or event into labeled white envelopes or photo storage boxes separated by dividers.

- Keep only those photos worth keeping. Poor-quality photos or boring shots (do you really need to keep all ten photos of the

CHATTER TIME

Kristin told her group how she and her husband actually scheduled a photo-organizing weekend after feeling guilty that more than eight years of photographs (since their wedding) had been just thrown into one big unorganized basket. She arranged for her children to visit their grandmother for the weekend so she and her husband had two full, uninterrupted days specifically earmarked for photo organizing. Kristin admits it took them longer than she had anticipated because it was hard not to stop and reminisce at all the memories in hand. It proved to be not only a meaningful activity for them as a couple, but an efficient way to quickly get a grip on all the photo clutter she had. Her photos are now either in albums, displayed in frames, or sorted and stored properly.

same sunset?) should be tossed. You might want to use some of your duplicate photos as gifts to other people.

- Store all photographs upright in the photo boxes along with their negatives. Label the boxes by year or occasion. Keep the boxes in a cool dry place such as a closet where the temperature will not be too hot or too cold, rather than in your attic, where heat may cause fading, or in your basement, where moisture can encourage mold.

- If you have a computer, check into the various systems now on the market for storing photographs digitally. Many film processors can burn your favorite photos onto a CD for a small fee. Or you can use a home scanner.

ALBUMS AND FRAMES

- When your photographs are sorted and labeled by month and year, you are ready to begin organizing them in photo albums or scrapbooks, or displaying them in frames.

- Gather your supplies: scissors, glue sticks or mounting corners, a small paper cutter (many craft stores have small cutters specifically designed for cropping photos), colored craft paper (even wrapping paper) for colorful photo backdrops on the album pages, pens/markers, photo boxes, albums, assorted picture frames, and even a basket of novelty sticker designs to brighten up photo album pages.

- Do not use old magnetic photo albums made with Mylar or PVC (polyvinyl chloride). Both will accelerate deterioration. They have a very high acidic content and can start eating through your photographs in about fifteen years.

- If you haven't been putting photos into albums for years, the easiest way to get started is to work on an album with your most recent photos and continue backward from there. Sometimes a helpful way to begin is creating theme albums, such as a holiday album to encompass your holiday photos from the past several years.

- Don't use every photo for the pages of your albums; select a few that best represent a specific occasion. You can store the rest in your photo boxes.
- Crop each photo as you see fit. You can fit more photos onto one page if they are cropped. For instance, if you are displaying a photo of your parents in the backyard, do you really need to include all of the blue sky that takes up a third of the photo? Crop it down. Don't, however, crop away all backgrounds. Some backgrounds are integral parts of your memories . . . your childhood home or the old tire swing hanging from the weeping willow tree in the backyard. Keeping some background can also help with size distinction; your toddler standing next to the mailbox, for instance, marks his height at a glance.
- Make a point to pull out and collect those one-of-a-kind prize photographs you know you will cherish always. Enlarge them for decorative photo frames or display them all together in a family photo album to be kept out on the coffee table.
- Create a yearly collage of photos. Each year, purchase a collage mat with various shaped cutouts to insert photos into, and keep it hanging near your home desk. Throughout the year, as that certain special photo comes into your home, add it to the collage. Frame the mat when completed and create a display wall for your collages in a stairwell or the family room.
- Never display a colored photo in direct sunlight. Once the color dyes fade, the photo cannot be restored.
- Start a birthday theme album for each of your kids. Use two pages for each birthday: the first page for an enlarged photo of your child on that day, and the second page for a few assorted pictures of his or her birthday party.
- Consider creating a family heirloom album. Collect old photo-

graphs from your ancestry (copy them at a copy store if you are
borrowing photos from relatives). Don't forget to add captions
with names of people, explanations, or stories about the
photos.

- Keep a travel album for revisiting favorite trips at a glance.
- Put together a goodnight album. One grandmother told us she
keeps a family album in the guest room where her small grand-
son sleeps when he visits. She uses the album at bedtime to
share stories with him about when his daddy was a little boy.
- Keep collecting all those yearly holiday photo cards you don't
know what to do with. Put them into a big photo album you can
label "friends and family," so they will be organized and allow
you to experience things like watching your college roommate's
kids grow up.
- Publish your family history! A company called 1stBooks Library
can actually publish your family photos and historical memoirs
as a bookstore quality book. A great gift for a family member or
an excellent coffee table book! Visit www.1stbooks.com.

The Key: Attaching This Step to Your Current Lifestyle

- Get into the habit of sorting and putting away every packet of
photos as soon as you bring them into your home. One package
should take you less than ten minutes.
- When going on your biannual yard sale adventures, start looking for unique photo frames. Having proper display cases on
hand is a big part of updating your photo maintenance.
- Keeping photos organized can be an ongoing family time craft
project to do together after school or on weekends.
- Start regular photo-organizing/scrapbook dates with friends or

family members who also need to get their photos organized.
Every Wednesday morning, for instance, after the kids get off to
school, you'll look forward to the coffee and photo-organizing
time with friends.

· If you find your own unique way to attach this step to your personal lifestyle, please share your ideas with us on our Web site:
www.SimpleStepsProgram.com.

Gratitude Journal

Keep a Daily Gratitude Journal

Why Should We Keep a Gratitude Journal?

- Writing in a gratitude journal gives us a happy, grateful spirit.
- A grateful spirit brightens our mood, boosts our energy, and infuses our daily living with a sense of joyful abundance. Dianne Hales wrote in "The Gratitude Diet" in *Ladies' Home Journal*, "The meek may inherit the Earth, but the grateful most enjoy their days upon it."
- A gratitude journal helps us focus on the simple, everyday things that make our lives even just a little bit better.
- It certainly isn't easy to be grateful all the time. We all have our days. But just knowing that you are going to write in your gratitude journal will help you look at your day differently.
- Beginning or ending each day with joyful entries in a journal forces us to acknowledge the positive in each day and in our lives.
- Training ourselves to think positively is one of the best ways to improve our emotional health.
- Keeping a gratitude journal encourages us to be thankful for our friends and families, our health, our home, even our bodies

and the way we look. As a result, we say thank you more often, extend kind gestures more often, and accept compliments more appreciatively.

· Gratitude has a cleansing effect on the soul, healing us from the inside out, says writer Marianne Williamson. She tells us that saying thank you is an act of spiritual power.

How to Keep a Daily Gratitude Journal

· You can use any type of journal: a blank hardcover bound journal, your daily planner, a spiral notebook, a pad of paper, your digital assistant, or even space beside your meal entries in your current food journal.

· Starting today, write three things you are grateful for.

· Try not to just repeat gratitude for your children and spouse on a daily basis. Look to the broader world.

· Make your daily entries about things you have experienced that day—different things that moved you, touched you in some way and brightened your outlook, or something that brought you joy that day, no matter how big or how small.

· Oprah Winfrey once told us at a motivational seminar in Chicago that if she ever got stuck thinking of a gratitude entry, she would simply write "breathing." Be grateful for the simple fact that you are here, alive and well.

· You may say thank you for the obvious big gifts that come your way each day: a job promotion, a new car, another pound lost, or good news from your doctor. But don't forget to say thank you for the smaller, more subtle gifts that pass through your day: the baby birds you notice in a nest outside your window, having just enough milk left for your favorite morning cereal, or the stain that finally lifted from your favorite blouse.

- And perhaps you should also say thank you on those particular days where a gift might be wrapped in heartache. Learn to say thank you in times of adversity because a gift may take the form of a life lesson, even if you cannot see it yet.
- If you've recently experienced tragedy or sorrow and find it difficult to begin a gratitude journal, Laura King, Ph.D., suggests these steps: First, step back from your disappointment. For three days in a row, write for ten minutes about what you've learned from the negative experience. Finally, decide you want a happy ending and try to make the dream a reality. "We are our life stories," King says. "The way that story ends is really important."
- On those days you consider especially challenging, you should try to list even more than three gratitude entries. This forces you to look beyond any difficulties.
- After several weeks of writing three entries, try working up to five gratitude entries daily.

The Key: Attaching This Step to Your Current Lifestyle

- Try to write in your gratitude journal at the same time and place each day, so it becomes a normal part of your day.
- Every night, get into the habit of taking a moment to reflect upon your day. Leave your gratitude journal with a pen on your nightstand to serve as a reminder to jot down your entries before bed.
- Make thankfulness a part of your day. After getting dressed each morning, look at yourself in a full-length mirror and give yourself a compliment. Why not add a compliment to yourself as an extra daily gratitude journal entry?

- Challenge yourself. Make it a habit to give at least one compliment before you reach your office door in the morning. Perhaps it was to the building doorman who lost some weight, or the parking lot attendant's new hairstyle, or on your daughter's choice of a blouse that morning.
- Go the extra mile with gratitude. Don't just say thank you in your journal but try to express gratitude throughout your day. Compliment your dry cleaner for the nice work they've been doing, buy lunch for a coworker who helped you meet an important deadline, or pick some garden flowers for your daughter's piano teacher. Extending gratitude every day assists you with finding entries for your daily journal.
- At the dinner table, make an evening family ritual of everyone listing the best two things that happened to them that day.
- Each night, when you tuck your children into bed, share verbal gratitude entries together. This is a fun way for your children to cultivate an appreciative attitude in life.
- Keeping a gratitude journal makes grateful people. And perhaps, most important, the benefit of being a grateful person is the ability to spread your generosity to others. Generosity is contagious. Smile at a stranger, compliment the grocery checkout clerk, or wink at your husband as he's taking out the garbage. You are allowing someone else to taste the sweetness of a grateful moment.
- Make it easier each day to find things to be grateful for. Consider doing volunteer work in your local community. When you see others who may not be as fortunate, it helps you appreciate the things you have. Whether you volunteer for a local charity, help at a school, or visit a nursing home, the simple act of giving your time establishes a link between yourself and others, helps make the world a better place, and brings more fulfill-

ment to your own life. For more information on volunteering, log on to www.independentsector.org.

- If you find your own unique way to attach this step to your personal lifestyle, please share your ideas with us on our Web site: www.SimpleStepsProgram.com.

Sharing

Iris Finds a New Sense of Freedom
on the Simple Steps Program

At the age of seventy-two, Iris, a native of England, has found a new lease on life after completing the Simple Steps ten-week plan several times over!

"I followed the program initially to learn how to eat better and lose some weight," she recalls. In retrospect, she now realizes that she was actually looking for a lifeline that she didn't know she needed.

"I was in such a rut," she explains in her soft English accent. "I had so many losses over three years. I lost my mother. I lost a good friend. I lost a job that I had and I lost a business I tried to start. It was just one thing after another. I gained weight and I wasn't doing anything to help myself. I was sort of sinking."

Her family and her faith, along with the new circle of friends she met through her Simple Steps workshop, helped her climb out of that rut. The retired wife and mother started feeling brighter and happier after the very first meeting. "I think because it was such a friendly circle of people. Everyone seemed to have something to say. I didn't feel so alone. I realized that other people had their own situations to deal with. I was inspired by their stories, and grateful that the group was so positively charged."

As the weeks went by, Iris started dropping weight. She started feeling better about herself. She would never miss a meeting. In one winter morning's snow flurry, Iris' car wouldn't make it up the hill to where our meetings were held. In her seventies, Iris trudged up the snow-covered road on foot! She was determined. The new Iris was emerging.

Iris did have some roadblocks, but she learned how to work around them. With her arthritis, she found it painful to do her walking assignment each week, so she would walk in shorter spurts and expand upon her daily stretching for her primary physical exercise. During her first ten weeks on Simple Steps she got bad news from her doctor. Not only had arthritis set into her knees, but she now had a mild heart condition to contend with. "I think if I had heard the news before I started this program, it would have pulled me under even further. But because I had support and renewed energy, I was able to just push through it."

Working on weekly de-cluttering projects in her home has kept Iris active and kept her mind on something productive. It seems to have paid off. After the first ten weeks, Iris lost 28 pounds. When she repeated the program another time, a couple of old Simple Steps pals almost didn't recognize her. "Iris looks fabulous!" said one woman after the meeting. "She looks so much younger, so radiant." Today, Iris has lost a total of 40 pounds. "I still have more weight to lose," she says. "I would like to lose another 50 pounds. But everybody sees the difference. My son in England was amazed when I went to visit him. And my husband has been totally supportive."

Iris is convinced that the whole experience is about so much more than losing weight, her original goal. "I look at my desk now. It's lovely and tidy. I've met a great group of women from all walks of life. I now know you can pick yourself up. I'm so grateful."

Iris expressed her gratitude to the founders of the Simple Steps program by writing a special thank-you card. "I feel like the girl on the card!" she wrote of the young girl pictured on the front, smiling with arms stretched to the sky. "Free! Free of clutter, free of guilt, and free of unwanted pounds. A world of thanks to you!"

Now Iris' card has a special place in the founding authors' Simple Steps gratitude journal. The ripple effect. Gratitude is contagious.

Congratulations!

You've now mastered the following Simple Steps. Read them aloud as a positive affirmation. Make them a habit and keep them up as part of your new lifestyle.

I am drinking eight cups of water daily

I am walking twenty minutes a day

I am clearing out one drawer/cabinet/closet space every week

I am saving $2 a day (or 1 percent of my weekly salary)

I am keeping a daily food journal

I am squeezing in some isometrics every day

I am maintaining an efficient laundry system

I am following a daily to-do list

I am taking a multivitamin every day

I am aware of my posture and breathing

I am keeping a clear desktop

I am cleansing and moisturizing daily

I am replacing bad fats with good fats

I am dancing to at least one song every day

I am maintaining a clean and healthy refrigerator and pantry

I am cleaning and flossing my teeth twice daily

I am cutting back on caffeine

I am discovering the benefits of yoga

I am maintaining a system to avoid mail piles

I am finding daily serenity time

I am replacing processed foods with whole grains

I am doing a few minutes of crunches every day

I am maintaining a clean car

I am dressing smart and keeping my closet organized

I am eating more slowly, respecting food

I am greeting the day with morning stretches

I am organizing my photos

I am keeping a gratitude journal

The Evening Primrose

Delicate and subtle,
a determined soul.
A free spirit.

No Night Eating

Do Not Eat at Least Two Hours Before Going to Bed

Why Should We Stop Eating Two Hours Before Bed?

- Our bodies need approximately twelve hours for our digestive and circulatory systems to rest. (That's why our morning meal is called breakfast—breaking the fast.)
- Our research shows that if we avoid night eating, we wake up feeling better and less bloated. When we snack late at night, we are more likely to wake up with a junk food hangover.
- Heavy meals late at night leave us gassy and bloated. They can also cause us to feel overtired, since our body needs even more energy to digest the food.
- A large meal, especially one containing carbohydrates, before we go to bed stimulates insulin, which in turn stimulates fat storage and prevents fat burning. An easy way to lose weight is to stop eating as early in the evening as possible. Try not eating after seven p.m. and see what happens.

WEIGHT LOSS TIP

Practicing this simple step is vital and should become a lifestyle habit if you are trying to lose weight. If you snack in the evenings, following this step alone should help you take off pounds quickly.

How to Curb Night Eating

· Adjust your dinnertime if necessary. If you hold off dinner because you wait for your spouse to get home, stop! You should eat earlier and then when he gets home sit with him with a cup of herbal tea and conversation.

· If you typically get home from work late, try eating a larger lunch during the day to keep hunger under control and have a light dinner when you come home.

· Watch the portion sizes and calories you consume at dinner. Your lightest meal should be in the evening. By early afternoon, more than half of your day's calories should have already been consumed.

· Don't skip breakfast or lunch.

· For dinner, choose foods that are easy to digest. Try vegetables, fruits, and small amounts of starches, advises Terri Brownlee, nutrition director of Duke University's Diet and Fitness Center.

· Beware of mindless eating (such as in front of the TV). Night snacking is usually not hunger related.

· Research has found that we consume more calories in low to dim light (for example, in front of the TV or in a mood-set restaurant), because we are much less self-conscious. So if you're watching calories, turn up the lights.

- Set a deadline for yourself that works with your lifestyle. Do you eat at seven-thirty p.m. and go to bed at ten p.m.? Then no eating after eight p.m.!

WEIGHT LOSS TIP

Whatever you crave in the evening, allow yourself to have it the next morning. You won't feel deprived and will have the whole next day to burn the calories . . . and you may not want it the next day!

The Key: Attaching This Step to Your Current Lifestyle

- Make a rule to never eat in your family room.
- Use willpower. Keep busy with your hands at night by knitting, reading, folding clothes, or playing games with your kids. Dis-associate television from snacking.
- Instead of getting dessert, brew a pot of herbal tea. Sip the tea throughout the evening.
- Go for a walk after dinner to start the digestive process.
- Start a creative project and get into the habit of working on it for an hour or so every evening after dinner. Take up painting or pottery, or work on a de-clutter project. Simply getting up from the dinner table and being active helps you refocus your thoughts away from mindless snacking.

- Paint your nails after dinner to keep you from reaching for a snack.
- Every time you crave a late-night snack, put 25 cents in a jar. At the end of the month, treat yourself to a movie night or better yet, donate the money to a homeless shelter.
- The next time you think you're hungry, drink a big glass of water. Often we're dehydrated, not hungry.
- If you find your own unique way to attach this step to your personal lifestyle, please share your ideas with us on our Web site: www.SimpleStepsProgram.com.

Strength Training

Add Strength Training Exercises to Your Fitness Routine Each Week

Why Do We Need Strength Training?

- Strength training tones muscles and improves endurance.
- In addition to increasing muscle mass, strength training also improves balance, posture, and alignment and helps burn off extra calories. For every pound of muscle we create, our body burns 30 to 40 more calories a day, and that's just at rest, according to *Self* magazine, March 2002. In comparison, one pound of fat burns off only 2 calories when we're at rest.
- Strength training can make us look leaner and we may drop a few dress sizes, even if we haven't lost any weight.
- Weight-bearing exercise fights osteoporosis.
- Strength training enhances self-esteem and self-confidence.
- Strength training will increase the quality of our sleep, says Dr. Miriam Nelson, professor at the School of Nutrition Science and Policy at Tufts University and author of *Strong Women Eat Well*.
- It's never too late to start a workout program. Twenty women of postmenopausal age participated in a study that required them to begin a strength training program. After doing a five-

exercise workout twice a week for one year, the women were in the same physical condition as women fifteen to twenty years younger, according to Dr. Nelson.

· Muscles serve as shock absorbers, so strengthening them may help keep injuries at bay.

· Don't forget, strength training tones all of our muscles, including our heart. It lowers our resting heart rate, which makes our heart work more efficiently.

How to Strength Train

· Strength train only two or three days a week.

· Never exercise the same muscles two days in a row.

· Warm up before starting. Following your daily walk would be a good time to strength train, or do five minutes of jumping jacks and stretching without weights before you begin training.

· For an exercise requiring weights, start slowly by using a pair of light hand weights (3 to 5 pounds). Starting out too heavy or too fast may discourage you. This is a life commitment, so work at your own pace and build from there.

· To choose the right hand weights for yourself, lift a hand weight eight times. If you can't lift it by the seventh or eighth time during the first set, then it's too heavy. Make sure the weight feels comfortable to you.

· Start with one weekly session of various weight-bearing exercises. Do three sets of eight repetitions of each exercise. As your ability increases, you can move up to three sets of ten to twelve repetitions.

· Watch yourself while you train. Find a spot in front of a mirror and watch to be sure you are doing the exercise correctly and your posture is correct; your back, neck, and head should be straight and in-line to prevent muscle injury. Watch your wrists; they should be straight, not bent in any direction.

· Remember to breathe. *Exhale when resistance is coming toward your body and inhale when moving weights away from your body.*

· If you are in any pain, stop. You may be doing the exercise wrong, or the weight may be too heavy.

· Wear comfortable clothing and a good pair of athletic shoes while you train.

· Make sure to stretch all muscles that you have worked. Strength training shortens your muscles, so you need to stretch them back out. Stretching also eases sore muscles. (For more information on stretching, see Simple Step 26.)

SIMPLE STRENGTH TRAINING EXERCISES

To help prevent wiggly arms and legs, below are a few strength training exercises you can try. Choose two or three to get you started, making sure to focus on a different muscle group for each exercise.

SQUAT (HIPS, BUTTOCKS, AND INNER THIGHS):
Stand with your feet hip width apart and toes pointing forward. Grasp a hand weight in each hand, your palms facing your thighs and out in front of you. With your back straight, head up, and looking forward, slowly bend your knees as if to sit down. Keep knees and ankles

aligned as you lower yourself into a seated position (you should not feel any pain). Slowly straighten your knees to the starting position. If you are a beginner, you can try this one without the weights and work your way up.

LUNGE (HIPS, BUTTOCKS, AND INNER THIGHS):

Stand with your feet hip width apart and your arms down. Grip weights in your hands, with palms toward your thighs. Contract your abdominal muscles through-out the entire set. Step forward with your left foot, bending both knees. Your left knee should be directly above your toes. Keep your back straight. Sink down so your left thigh is parallel to the floor for a slow count of five. Do not touch your right knee to the floor, and keep your arms down alongside your thighs. Return to the starting position; repeat with your other leg.

TRICEPS PUSH-UP (TRICEPS AND SHOULDERS):

Lie with your stomach on the floor. Keeping your knees on the floor, pick up your feet and cross them. Put your hands on the floor and keep them tightly by your upper ribs. Push up off the ground, keeping your back and neck in a straight line and your abs con-tracted at all times (you do not want an arch or curve in your back). Lower your torso again, so that your chest almost touches the floor. For beginners, you can try

push-ups by standing parallel to and a couple feet
away from a wall and pushing up from the wall.

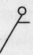

SHOULDER PRESSES (TRICEPS AND SHOULDERS):

Stand or sit on a chair. Holding a hand weight in each
hand, start with your elbows tucked in at each side of
your waist and your hands by your shoulders, palms
facing forward. Keeping your back straight and your
abdomenal muscles tight, slowly straighten your arms
up and raise the hand weights over your head, bringing them together once your arms are fully extended.
Slowly bring them back down to starting position.
Repeat.

BENT-OVER ROW (UPPER BODY AND BACK):

Using a hand weight of 3 to 5 pounds, grip one weight
in your right hand. With a workout bench or bed to
your left, bend your left leg at the knee and rest your
shin flat on the surface. Lean forward at the hips so
your head and neck are in line with your spine. Keeping your back straight, rest the palm of your left hand
on the bed above your knee, directly under your left
shoulder. Lower your right arm straight to the ground,
palm facing the bed. Pull up, keeping your elbows
close to your body, until your right hand is even with
your ribs, squeeze your shoulder blades together,
then lower back down to the starting position.

BICEP CURL (BICEPS):
Stand with your feet shoulder width apart, knees slightly bent, and toes straight ahead. Hold 3- to 8-pound hand weights with an underhand grip (palms facing the ceiling). Relax shoulders, which should be down and back. Look straight ahead. Starting with the weights at waist level, lift weights up toward chest, keeping your elbows directly below your shoulders and close to your waist. Make sure to keep your wrists straight. Pause, and then slowly return to the starting position. Repeat.

The Key: Attaching This Step to Your Current Lifestyle

- You should strength train two or three days a week, allowing a rest day in between. Pick the best hour of day for you, and then do it at the same hour always.
- Keep a hand weight at your desk, so you can pick up the weight and lift while on the phone.
- Get your walking partner or spouse to strength train with you to help you keep the habit.
- Keep weights in the kitchen so you can do some reps in between steps of making dinner.
- Skip dessert on Tuesdays and Thursdays and replace it with an after-dinner strength training session.

CHITCHAT

Don't let muscle soreness be a deterrent to continuing your strength training program. I remember when I started strength training, I was painfully sore the next day (and for a few days afterward), but friends who also worked out assured me it was a "good" sore. I didn't see at that time how what I was feeling could be considered "good"; I felt pain and didn't want to do anything! But now that I strength train at least three days a week for twenty to thirty minutes, when I ache, I know it as a "good" sore. I also know that I have to stretch and work out that soreness. Strength training is so important to all of us and to our health; I wish you all the best in your journey—it truly is worth the weight.

—Linda McClintock

- Do strength training exercise while you watch TV.
- If you find your own unique way to attach this step to your personal lifestyle, please share your ideas with us on our Web site: www.SimpleStepsProgram.com.

Your Bed

Make Your Bed Every Day

Why Should We Make Our Bed?

- Our mood and outlook for the entire day is largely determined by how we encounter the first few waking minutes. It feels good to start our day with instant tidiness. Keeping our bed neat and organized is an easy way to do this.
- What takes just a moment of time can start off a day full of organization.
- Our bed is the focal point of the room; an unmade bed creates an unorganized bedroom. With minimum effort, we should keep the bedroom a relaxing and comfortable haven for us to enjoy. A messy bed can end up being an energy drain that creates laziness and deters us from cleaning up anything else in the room.
- By making our bed daily, we are more apt to pay attention to the condition of our bed linens and be more disciplined with washing and changing the sheets every week.
- A tidy bed will help us sleep better. Making our bed creates a peaceful place to sleep. There are few such wonderful and calming things as slipping into crisp linens at the end of the day.

How to Take Care of Your Bed

- Purchase a mattress pad to cover and protect the mattress from spills, staining, and everyday wear and tear.
- Beginning at the top corner of your bed, place the bottom fitted sheet into place. Align the flat sheet on top of the fitted sheet with the right side down, so when you fold it over the blanket you can see the design. Tuck the flat sheet into the mattress. Pleat the corners and tuck in for a crisp, neat finish.
- Properly cared for, sheets should last three to five years. We suggest finding sheets with a thread count of at least 200 in 100 percent cotton. For a noticeably softer sheet, you may consider Egyptian cotton, which contains long fibers that will not pill or lint.
- Top the sheet with a blanket or comforter, depending on the season. Use a blanket with a bedspread or quilt for extra warmth.
- When making your bed, don't forget to clean your headboard. Brighten brass, revive wood finishes, and even vacuum or dust wicker weaves.
- You may choose to hide any exposed metal supports or bed rails with a bed skirt or dust ruffle, available at most linen outlets or department stores.
- To keep pillows clean and fresh, zip pillows into protective, washable covers, or use two pillowcases for each pillow; the open end of the first case should go into the covering case.
- Test your pillow; an old, floppy one does not provide the necessary support for your head, neck, and spinal cord and can lead to pain, stiffness, and restless sleep. To check your pillow, fold it in half. If it doesn't open back up again on its own, it's time for a new one, says James Maas, Ph.D., author of *Power Sleep*.
- Don't overpillow your bed with too many decorative throw pil-

lows. One accent pillow in an interesting shape or color can make a classic design statement without cluttering your bed.

- To rinse out detergent buildup and make your sheets and pillowcases smell super clean, add ½ cup baking soda to the wash water. Many of the new linen sprays will keep your sheets sweet smelling between laundering.

- Fluff your pillows and comforter monthly by placing them in the dryer with a sheet of fabric softener. Tumble on the air-only setting for twenty minutes.

- Don't forget to launder your comforter, if your washing machine has the capacity to hold it, or send it out to be done. If it needs to be dry-cleaned, send it out seasonally.

- Be sure to flip your mattress every one to three months—side to side the first time, then head to toe the next. Vacuum it at least once a month with the upholstery brush attachment on your vacuum. Use an upholstery shampoo to remove any dirt or stains.

- If you use the space under your bed for storage, remove the containers twice a year, vacuum the carpet, and clean the containers before you put them back.

- If you tend to gather a lot of bed clutter, try using decorative baskets nearby to organize discarded clothing, books, and magazines that usually wind up tossed on your bed.

- Hang extra bedspreads or blankets on hangers in the back of your clothes closet or on a rod on the back of your bedroom door, so they're easily accessible when you need them.

The Key: Attaching This Step
to Your Current Lifestyle

- As soon as you get out of bed, get into the habit of turning around and making it.
- If this step is a new habit for you, post a little note near your toothbrush holder reminding you, "Don't forget, make your bed!" As soon as you rinse your teeth, head back into your room and make the bed.
- Be a kid again and try the reward system. Hang a small calendar by your nightstand and place a star on each day that you make your bed. Seeing that alone should serve as a reminder of your new habit.
- Make your bed while you watch your morning news show or just before you weight train.
- If you find your own unique way to attach this step to your personal lifestyle, please share your ideas with us on our Web site: www.SimpleStepsProgram.com.

Sleep

Get at Least One-half Hour More Sleep Every Night

Why Do We Need More Sleep?

- According to the Better Sleep Council, average adults require a minimum of seven or eight hours of sleep nightly.
- Inadequate sleep results in stress, lower motivation, and slower reflexes. The National Commission on Sleep Disorders Research estimates that insufficient sleep costs billions of dollars annually in traffic and industrial accidents.
- Chronic sleep debt hampers the body's ability to process carbohydrates. This causes our body to store more fat, according to an article in *Runner's World* magazine, October 2001.
- Medical reports published in *Journal of the American Medical Association* in the summer of 2000 indicate that our REM (rapid eye movement) sleep stage (our dream stage) is most important. This is the only time our body actually stops *growing*. Our cells lie completely dormant, thus slowing the aging process. The best way to get more REM sleep is simply to get more sleep, because it occurs several times throughout the night.
- During sleep, our body secretes melatonin, cortisol, and other hormones to help repair old cells and burn fat, according to

Sonia Ancoli-Israel, Ph.D. at the University of California, San Diego.

· During deep sleep, organs, bones, and tissues are repaired, while during REM, emotions and memories are processed.

· Insufficient sleep can shorten our life. A University of Chicago study found that when test subjects seventeen to twenty-eight years old were restricted to four hours of sleep six nights in a row, their levels of hypertension, diabetes, and memory problems rose to levels associated with sixty-year-olds.

· When we are overtired, we tend to make poor food choices. These poor choices can lead to weight gain.

How to Get More Sleep

· Make sleep a priority. Don't put it aside for one more chore or another television show. Remember, it's important.

· Sleep on a good bed. Your mattress and foundation should not be too small, too soft, too hard, or too old. You need to be comfortable in order to sleep well.

· Cool bedrooms, white noise, and sleeping masks are all helpful in getting enough quality sleep. The ideal temperature to sleep in is 60 to 65 degrees. A room that's too hot or too cold can disturb your sleep.

· A dark room is most conducive for sleeping. Light is a powerful time cue to our bodies, so try to block out light that might be sneaking in through thin curtains and cracks.

· Don't watch television in bed. The noise and light increase your alertness and make it difficult to sleep.

· Don't go to bed with a full stomach, because it can be harder to fall asleep.

· Refrain from consuming acidic foods in the evening, such as

orange juice, tomato sauce, or spicy dishes, as they may cause
heartburn, which can disrupt sleep.

· Avoid stimulants within three to six hours of bedtime. Stimulants affect deep sleep and can increase nighttime awakenings,
as declared by the Better Sleep Council. Cigarettes are a stimulant, and smokers have a harder time falling asleep than non-
smokers and don't get as much deep sleep. Drinking beverages
containing caffeine in the evening can also make it difficult to
fall asleep and stay in a deep sleep through the night.

· Avoid drinking alcohol at night as well. Although alcohol might
make you fall asleep faster, the sleep does not usually last
through the night.

· Sip a natural relaxant such as warm milk to induce sleep. A
warm glass of milk contains tryptophan—a chemical that makes
you sleepy.

The Key: Attaching This Step to Your Current Lifestyle

· Keep regular hours even on the weekends. Go to bed and get up
at the same time.

· Develop a sleep ritual so your body will be cued to settle down
for the night. Perhaps reading or listening to soothing music
will help you relax.

· If you have had an especially trying day, journal your thoughts
at least one hour before getting into bed to release any tension
you may be holding.

· Read something inspirational or uplifting just before bed so
that you enter a sleep state with a good frame of mind.

· Regular exercise should help. According to a Stanford University study published in *Journal of the American Medical Associa-*

tion, those who exercised a minimum of four and a half hours a week fell asleep twice as quickly—twelve minutes faster—and slept almost an hour longer than sedentary people.

- Soak in a hot tub before bed. The water temperature should be about 104 degrees and you should soak for approximately thirty minutes. For an extra indulgence, add soothing lavender oil to the water. While soaking, play calming music and turn down the lights. A candlelit bath is always relaxing.
- Wear socks to bed. A warm pair of socks causes blood vessels to dilate, lowering your core temperature and inducing sleep, according to a 1999 study published in *Nature* magazine.
- Dim the lights after nine p.m. to help cue your body into its sleep mode.
- If you find your own unique way to attach this step to your personal lifestyle, please share your ideas with us on our Web site: www.SimpleStepsProgram.com.

Sharing

Lois Turns the Clock Back and
Regains Her Youthful Lifestyle!

The Simple Steps program proved to be much more than Lois expected. She entered the workshop looking for diet and de-clutter tips and walked away with a new outlook on life. "It went way beyond dieting and de-cluttering; I tapped into my spiritual being and found more balance in all aspects of my life."

Simple Steps helped Lois deal with her sometimes hectic schedule. "Instead of becoming overwhelmed, I learned how to divide my time into small chunks and go back to a particular de-clutter or diet step and focus on that one. Sometimes I would take a walk or get on my exercise bike just to take a breather and think."

"I could always diet and lose weight when I was younger," Lois recalls. "It was always quick and effortless. Then what happened? Suddenly every pound becomes such a chore. And every time I lost weight, I gained it back. I must have lost and gained a hundred pounds over the years." But Lois did finally manage to break her weight plateau through the Simple Steps program. She lost 12 pounds in ten weeks, and although she admits she'd still like to lose another 10 pounds, she is happier, motivated, feeling younger, and refocused now.

Lois is a caretaker by nature. She has been married for thirteen years, and works as a speech pathologist for the school system and a home health agency. "I work with many women. I belong to several women's groups, an investment club, and a book club. But there was something so different about all the women I met through the Simple Steps program. We connected on such a deeper level. We were all there sharing our souls and truly inspiring each other."

The support of other women was just one unique part of the program. "One week, discussing gratitude, we were to send someone a secret compliment. How great is that! I think about that often. We should all show more gratitude."

Lois believes the steps she learned from the program are now healthy habits for life. "I have never in the past been able to stick to a diet while I was on vacation. Just recently, I spent some time vacationing in Kennebunkport, Maine, and stayed active and focused on good and healthy things. It's because the Simple Steps program teaches you a way of life. It's not a diet. I'm hooked on so many good new habits. I feel wonderful."

Even the space around Lois has become organized. She is proud to claim that everything she de-cluttered and organized at her home during the program is still exactly the same. She vows never to go back to her old ways. "I'm about to start my basement," she says on her way down to a project she had been putting off for a long time. She'll take it one garbage bag at a time.

Anything is possible. Just ask Lois. She feels she's captured a piece of her youth forever. "I feel great. Everyone should take the Simple Steps path."

Lois is now beginning to take steps toward one of her passions. As a speech therapist for people in need, and a lover of animals, she has decided to merge the two into a special care therapy, bringing pets into nursing homes and to children in hospitals.

Congratulations!

You've now mastered the following Simple Steps. Read them aloud as positive affirmation. Make them a habit and keep them up as part of your new lifestyle.

I am drinking eight cups of water daily

I am walking twenty minutes a day

I am clearing out one drawer/cabinet/closet space every week

I am saving $2 a day (or 1 percent of my weekly salary)

I am keeping a daily food journal

I am squeezing in some isometrics every day

I am maintaining an efficient laundry system

I am following a daily to-do list

I am taking a multivitamin every day

I am aware of my posture and breathing

I am keeping a clear desktop

I am cleansing and moisturizing daily

I am replacing bad fats with good fats

I am dancing to at least one song every day

I am maintaining a clean and healthy refrigerator and pantry

I am cleaning and flossing my teeth twice daily

I am cutting back on caffeine

I am discovering the benefits of yoga

I am maintaining a system to avoid mail piles

I am finding daily serenity time

I am replacing processed foods with whole grains

I am doing a few minutes of crunches every day

I am maintaining a clean car

I am dressing smart and keeping my closet organized

I am eating more slowly, respecting food

I am greeting the day with morning stretches

I am organizing my photos

I am keeping a gratitude journal

I am no longer eating at night

I am strength training each week

I am making my bed every morning

I am getting more sleep

The Pansy

*Joyful and colorful. Always smiling.
She loves life and brightens
the world with her presence.*

Spice Up Your Life

Find Creative Ways to Use Herbs and Spices

Why Should We Use Herbs and Spices?

- Spices add flavor to our meals without adding calories. When we reduce fat content in our meals, we can reduce the flavor. Spicing up bland food makes even vegetables more interesting.
- Using spices can sometimes rev up a slow metabolism. Research shows that we can increase our metabolism up to 25 percent by eating hot and spicy foods.
- Herbs and spices are a healthy alternative to salt. It's been proven in a recent government-sponsored DASH-Sodium study. Participants who kept their salt intake to 1,100 milligrams a day, ate a diet rich in produce and dairy, and replaced salt with herbs or spices such as pepper and basil reduced their systolic blood pressure by nine points in four weeks.
- Another use for herbs is aromatherapy. Oils scented with herbs can calm your nerves and add soothing scents to your life.
- A small window box or planting tray of fresh herbs and spices warms and decorates any kitchen.

HEALTH BENEFITS OF
HERBS AND SPICES

- *Chives* are one of the most well-known spices. Compounds in chives (part of the onion family) are believed to lower cholesterol and blood pressure, according to naturopathic doctor Mark Stengler, author of *The Natural Physician's Healing Therapies.* They are high in vitamin A, iron, calcium, and potassium. Using chives can also eliminate the need for salt.
- According to a USDA study, *oregano* packs a stronger antioxidant punch than oranges or apples. One tablespoon of fresh oregano delivers the same antioxidant dose as a medium-size apple. Oregano is a natural expectorant and can be used as a natural cough remedy.
- *Parsley* adds more than color to your plate. It is loaded with vitamin C, iron, and calcium. Parsley also acts as a diuretic and flushes out toxins along with excess fluid.
- *Garlic* reduces blood pressure and protects your heart. Researchers at New York Medical College in Valhalla reviewed evidence that showed that one-half to one clove daily of garlic lowered participants' blood pressure 9 percent after one month.
- *Basil* and *ginger* may be used to calm upset stomachs.
- *Ginger* acts as an anti-inflammatory agent. A study at Denmark's Odense University found that three-quarters of fifty-six participants with rheumatoid arthritis, osteoarthritis, or muscular pain got relief from both swelling and aches after taking ⅓ teaspoon ground ginger three times daily for at least three months.

- **Ginger** and **turmeric** have been found to destroy common bacteria such as salmonella, which causes food poisoning.
- **Cinnamon** may lower blood pressure, according to a new research study at George Washington University.

- Fresh herbs will not only fill our kitchen with bright, delicious scent but will add distinct flavor to our favorite dishes.

How to Use Spices and Herbs

- Visit your local library and take out a book on herbs and spices. Begin researching and experimenting with different herbs and spices.
- Many herbs are easy to grow—nothing tastes better than fresh herbs clipped from your garden.
- Herbs don't require much room to grow. You can plant an herb garden inside or outside.

COOKING WITH COMMON HERBS AND SPICES

- Don't cook fresh herbs. Add them to dishes at the last minute to preserve flavor.
- Using oil flavored with herbs and spices is a quick way to add flavor to a meal, and it is a healthier alternative to butter.
- Save calories by tossing greens with a tablespoon each of basil, parsley, and marjoram instead of dressing.
- Combine a can of tuna with herbs, a bit of olive oil, and lemon juice for a tasty salad without the mayonnaise.

- Lighten up your diet with a lean sauce for fish or poultry. Combine 2 tablespoons each of parsley, mint, and cilantro with 1 cup of nonfat plain yogurt. Stir in a chopped green onion.
- Use herbs and spices to coat meats before cooking rather than flour or bread coatings.
- Basil is a fine addition to most tomato dishes, soups, and salads. It is a mild, flavorful substitute for stronger spices such as garlic or pepper.
- Chives have a mild onion flavor and are great for dips.
- Use dill for salads, seafood, and dips.
- Parsley and thyme are welcome additions to salads, soups, or stir-fry dishes. Chop at the last minute—cooking parsley reduces its flavor and nutritional value.
- Rosemary and tarragon are great for seasoning grilled fish and chicken.
- Try fennel, mint, or chervil the next time you're cooking fish.
- Marjoram and savory spice up your rice and soups.
- Curry, paprika, and turmeric are good for color and add a zesty flavor to meats, salads, and stir-fry.
- Garlic adds a distinct flavor to most meals.
- Vanilla, cinnamon, and nutmeg are great for baking.

AROMATHERAPY: SPICING UP YOUR LIFE WITH HERBAL SCENTS

- Pamper yourself with the sweet smell of herbal oils. Get started on aromatherapy by purchasing 100 percent essential oils.
- Inhaling the aroma of peppermint oil can treat stomachaches, headaches, and congestion.
- The scent of chamomile oil is used to reduce indigestion, premenstrual syndrome, stress, and insomnia.
- Sweet-smelling lavender oil calms your nervous system.
- Make your own herbal pillow to help you sleep better. Tucked

STORING HERBS AND SPICES

DRIED

Store dried spices in airtight containers in a cool, dry place. Whole spices can last up to one year in airtight containers. Ground spices last a few months. The best way to check spices is to sniff and see if they are still aromatic. If they are not, they're too old. Purchase only small containers of herbs and spices unless you use them often.

FRESH

Store fresh herbal bouquets in your refrigerator in a glass of water. Cover them loosely with a plastic bag. Change water regularly and they will last for up to ten days. Ginger and chilies will stay fresh in the refrigerator for two to three weeks. It's a good idea to wrap ginger in paper towels or napkins to absorb moisture. Store chilies in a plastic bag. Stash lemongrass or curry leaves with a few drops of water in a sealed plastic bag in the crisper drawer.

FROZEN

Many fresh spices and herbs freeze well. Preserve herbs by washing and laying them flat on paper towels to dry. Place them in an airtight freezer bag and freeze. Freeze-dried whole herbs and spices have a shelf life of approximately one to two years. Peel spices such as ginger and freeze in a covered plastic container. Freeze lemongrass or curry for up to six months in airtight containers.

away inside a small pillow, herbs may help calm your nervous system and chase away sleeplessness, says Rosemary Gladstar, author of *Herbal Healing for Women*. To make a sleep pillow, fold an 8-inch piece of soft, appealing fabric in half. Sew two of the sides together inside out, leaving the third open for stuffing. Mix together the following dried herbs: 2 teaspoons of chamomile, 2 teaspoons of rose, and 2 teaspoons of lavender. Turn the pillow right side out and stuff the mixture inside. Sew the remaining side closed. Keep your sleep pillow beside your head or inside your pillowcase when you sleep. Fluff it a bit before you go to sleep to release the scent.

· Make your own potpourri sachets with fresh herbs. Pick herbs from your garden and dry them, either on a cookie sheet in the sun or by quick drying them in your oven on a cookie sheet at 100 degrees. Once they're dry, crush them and place them into a small sachet. Sachets can be made from your favorite mate-

---

WEIGHT LOSS TIP

If you are trying to lose weight, sprinkle some cayenne pepper on your food a couple times daily. Not only will you drink more water, but cayenne pepper raises your metabolism and body temperature, thereby releasing adrenaline, making you burn calories faster. In a research study conducted at Oxford Brookes University in England, dieters who added 1 teaspoon of cayenne pepper and 1 teaspoon of mustard to every meal raised their metabolism as much as 25 percent. The metabolism-raising effect of cayenne pepper can last up to five hours, says Marc Rogers, Ph.D., author of *Stuff Yourself Thin*.

rial, cheesecloth, or a coffee filter. Fill the sachet with herbs and either sew it closed or tie it closed with ribbon.

The Key: Attaching This Step to Your Current Lifestyle

- Visit the cookbook shelf at your local library or bookstore and try one of the many wonderful collections of recipes emphasizing herbs and spices.
- While grocery shopping each week, buy a different fresh herb to try cooking with.
- Get the family involved. Have your children pick sprigs of their favorite herbs and place them in fancy bottles with oil or vinegar. Label them and give as gifts.
- Put the saltshaker away. Take out the cayenne pepper and keep it right next to the black pepper.
- Spice up your life! Plant a window box in your kitchen and be sure to keep your scissors handy for fresh snips of herbs.
- Keep sachets in your clothes drawers, linen closet, car, clothes hamper, or wherever you want fresh sweet smells.
- If you find your own unique way to attach this step to your personal lifestyle, please share your ideas with us on our Web site: www.SimpleStepsProgram.com.

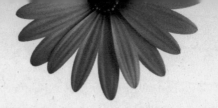

Cross-training

Add New Physical Activities Each Week

Why Should We Cross-train?

- Cross-training adds variety to our workout routine, fighting boredom.
- Cross-training helps our body stay in balance by working out more of our muscle groups. For instance, running one day uses our leg muscles, and swimming the next uses more upper-body muscles, while both exercises improve our cardiovascular system.
- Cross-training helps develop our entire body instead of just one area and thus may help reduce risk of injury.
- Cross-training increases endurance levels by making muscles stronger.
- By making us look leaner, cross-training improves our self-image.
- Changing our routine every day lets one part of our body rest while we're paying attention to another part.

How to Cross-train

- Choose different exercises—aerobic and nonaerobic—that you can do either daily or every other day, in addition to your twenty-minute walk. There are so many different indoor and outdoor activities you can try. If you think you may like to try a sport, go ahead—you probably will enjoy it. Try biking, swimming, playing ball, Pilates, yoga, or kayaking.
- Remember to choose opposite muscles for cross-training routines daily. One day work on your lower body (such as by jogging or biking) and the next work on your upper body (swimming or rowing).
- Find the right time of day to work out for your schedule. Start with twenty to thirty minutes every other day to get you in the habit of staying active. You may like it so much you will start working out every day, which would be better for you. Most trainers recommend at least one day of rest per week.
- Start at your own pace with each new exercise. As you continue, gradually increase length and intensity.
- Stretch every day for at least five to ten minutes, especially after each workout session.
- If you have lawn work to do, get outside and work in your yard. Raking, hoeing, moving rocks, and weeding can be a great part of your cross-training routine.
- Try cross-country skiing; it's great for your legs, torso, and arms.
- Go bicycling or jogging while your child is riding his or her bicycle next to you.
- Greet your children after school in your driveway. Jump rope, hop up and down on a pogo stick, shoot hoops, or play hopscotch with them.

BELOW IS A SAMPLE WEEK OF CROSS-TRAINING

- Monday: Ride your bike for thirty minutes and do upper-body weight training for twenty minutes.
- Tuesday: Swim laps for thirty minutes.
- Wednesday: Rollerblade for thirty minutes and do lower-body strength training for twenty minutes.
- Thursday: Try a fitness yoga tape or class for thirty minutes and take a second twenty-minute walk.
- Friday: Swim for thirty minutes.
- Saturday: Jog at your own pace for thirty minutes and do upper- and lower-body strength training for twenty minutes.
- Sunday: Take a family hike or family canoe trip.

- If you like to swim, find a pool in your community.
- Plan a vacation with cross-training in mind. Think about incorporating swimming, dancing, a bicycle tour, a hiking tour, or a canoe tour. Think variety!
- Try seasonal sports when weather is conducive, such as playing soccer out front with your kids, Rollerblading, surfing, tennis, and cross-country skiing.

The Key: Attaching This Step to Your Current Lifestyle

- Make an appointment for your health. Set up a cross-training routine. Mark your calendar and stick with it.
- Schedule a cross-training family day and try something new:

CHATTER TIME

Maureen, a participant in her fifties, always had a desire to Rollerblade. When cross-training was introduced as a Simple Step, she decided to go for it. Maureen practiced every evening after work in a local park. The guard at the park was so nervous watching Maureen that he actually moved to a different part of the park so he wouldn't have to witness any falls. Months later, as Maureen gracefully glided on her Rollerblades, she met up with the same guard. To her surprise, he was on Rollerblades, too. Maureen was curious what got him interested, and when she asked, he simply explained that if she could do it, *anyone* could! Maureen inspired him, and Rollerblading has become her favorite cross-training activity.

cross-country skiing, horseback riding, canoeing, hiking up a mountain, or just going outside and playing tag—anything that you think you'll enjoy.

· Try one new sport a month.

· Find a partner to experiment with you.

· Take a class to learn more about an activity you've been wanting to try.

· If you find your own unique way to attach this step to your personal lifestyle, please share your ideas with us on our Web site: www.SimpleStepsProgram.com.

Fix It

Do One Repair or Improvement Project Every Week

Why Do We Need to Fix It?

- Completing achievable repair or improvement projects simply makes us feel better; it makes us feel like we've accomplished something.
- Sometimes it's the little things that we keep putting off, such as replacing a lightbulb or fixing a leak, that drain our energy. Accomplishing quick fix-it projects such as sewing that loose button on our blouse or setting the clock on the VCR (that has been blinking 12:00 for years) makes us feel good.
- Each time we enter a room and we realize there's something needing attention, our focus is being disrupted and our concentration is being divided.
- If overlooked, these small projects or improvements can become overwhelming. If overwhelmed, we might never have the time or energy to fix or improve things around our home.
- Sooner or later the last of the four lightbulbs in our bathroom will go out, leaving us completely in the dark.
- If we don't take a few minutes to tighten the loose doorknobs, they will eventually fall off.

- Screens covering windows must be patched or replaced to prevent unwanted pests from entering our home.

CHATTER TIME

Gina's first fix-it list covered two entire pages of a notebook. As instructed, she transferred ten items from the notebook to her weekly to-do list. Each evening after work, Gina tackled a fix-it project on her list. She finished her first ten fix-it items before the to-be-completed date. Gina was energized by her accomplishments. Three months after she completed the Simple Steps program, we received a call from Gina. She was ecstatic and explained that for years, all these little fix-it projects had weighed her down. Previously, she had walked around her home as if with blinders on, because she was overwhelmed. Gina explained, "I have accomplished more in the past three months than I have in years. I am proud to report both pages of my original notebook list are complete. I have never felt better about my home or myself. Fix-it is now part of my lifestyle and I continue to create lists for all the little things before they overwhelm me."

How to Do Fix-It Projects and Improvements

- Approach fix-it projects with a can-do attitude.
- With a pen and notebook in hand, take a walking tour of your home. Walk from room to room making notes of all repairs or improvements that need to be done.
- While in each room, be sure to check from the ceiling to the floor for things you can improve upon.

- Once your list is complete, place projects into two categories: projects you can accomplish on your own and projects that require an expert to handle.
- If you have somebody who likes to tinker, perhaps you can seek his or her assistance for the projects you don't have time for or

---

FIX-IT IDEAS

- Sew buttons on with dental floss—it's much stronger than regular thread.
- Sharpen scissors by cutting through folded layers of foil wrap.
- Cover furniture scratches by filling them in with a matching colored marker.
- Fix small holes in screens with clear nail polish. Several coats might be necessary to fill in gaps.
- Use a potato or bar of soap to unscrew a broken lightbulb socket.
- To tighten loose drawer pulls, unscrew hardware, put a washer on the screw, and screw it back in.
- Lubricate nails or screws with a bit of soap to help make sinking them easier.
- To avoid hitting your thumb while hammering, stick the nail through a small piece of clay to hold it in place.
- When painting, pull an old pair of socks over your shoes to catch drippings.
- After painting a room, remember to keep a small jarful of that paint for touch-ups.

---

cannot accomplish alone, in exchange for some healthy baked goods or perhaps baby-sitting.

- Trade or switch projects with a neighbor or friend. For example, if you like to paint and your neighbor knows how to refinish furniture, swap projects.
- For matters that require expert attention, make a schedule and call the right person for the job to get things moving. Perhaps schedule one project a month to spread out expenses. You should record names and numbers of specialists you hear about who may be needed to handle future projects.
- The rest of the list is yours to tackle. Transfer eight to ten items to your weekly to-do lists. As you complete jobs on a weekly basis, add new ones.

The Key: Attaching This Step to Your Current Lifestyle

- Involve the family. Offer stars or points to be redeemed for movie passes, dinner at their favorite restaurant, or perhaps an ice cream sundae for family members who help you accomplish your list.
- Spend time with your significant other accomplishing projects together. Plan to spend an equal time together socially as an incentive.
- Reward yourself with a new outfit, manicure, or massage when your list is completed.
- If you find your own unique way to attach this step to your personal lifestyle, please share your ideas with us on our Web site: www.SimpleStepsProgram.com.

Passions

Rediscover Your Passions

Why Do We Need to Rediscover Our Passions?

- Our passions, those creative interests and hobbies we most enjoy—whether gardening, photography, piano, cooking, or golfing—are a big part of what defines each of us. Simply put, they're what make us who we are.
- Passions are nourishment for our soul. They keep us fulfilled.
- It is motivating to experience those activities or hobbies that have always brought us joy. They allow us to live with happiness and laughter on a daily basis.
- So many of us, especially women, seem to lose or give up our passions for caretaking roles. We tend to our children, our marriage, our home, and our work, but very often forget to tend to ourselves. It is important for us to rekindle the flames of our creative passions.
- Our passions can brighten up our days when we're feeling overwhelmed or troubled. They allow positive attitudes to shine through.

- Our passions provide a joyful outlet in a sometimes overscheduled day-to-day existence. They are a well-deserved break.
- To rediscover an old passion reconnects us with our youth. It keeps us young.
- Several years ago *60 Minutes,* on CBS, did a story on centenarians (people at least one hundred years old). The piece explored common factors these elderly men and women shared in the way they lived their lives. Quite surprisingly, it was not diet and exercise that appeared to keep these people going (after all, their generation was way before the oat bran craze), but rather a positive mental attitude, the ability to handle loss, and passions. Yes, passions! Having a hobby to be passionate about, to enjoy, to focus on, and to maintain mental agility seemed to be a common thread in living a long and satisfying life.
- Keeping up with our most passionate interests can pay off financially. Many of the most successful businesspeople in the world built their empires around things they were simply passionate about: Mrs. Fields loved baking cookies, Martha Stewart loved her home and garden, and Bill Gates was crazy for computers.

How to Rediscover a Lost Passion

- Make a list of your own favorite things. In addition to giving you pleasure, since this exercise is all about the things that please and excite you, listing your favorite things will also help you see what type of passions are really within you. Find them. Seek them out. Act on your passions today.
- Think about the things you enjoy doing most. Maybe there is one thing in particular that you have been thinking about. Now

that your kids are taking violin lessons, maybe you are yearning to start playing again.

- Once a month, as you write your gratitude entries into your journal, list one enjoyable pastime you would love to experience again. Or list a new one that you have yet to try.
- Keep a passion jar. Fill an empty jar with favorite items/events/ wishes written on various strips of different colored paper.

CHATTER TIME

Hannah, a young mother in one of our Simple Steps groups, admitted to us that her husband didn't know she had once been an accomplished classical pianist. "When we got married," she explained, "there were bills to pay. We both worked long hours to afford our home. We couldn't have afforded a piano, even if I wished for one. So I never said anything. Then came the babies and the daily grind of motherhood. It just seemed appropriate to go without my music. There were so many other things that took precedence." Hannah decided after completing the program that she wanted—she *needed*—to play piano again. She found a way. With permission from her minister, she was able to practice on an old piano in the church hall. She then invested in an electronic tabletop keyboard for playing at home. Her husband was amazed and so proud of her. Their children would sing to her music and put on fun family presentations. And just one year after completing her Simple Step assignment of rediscovering her passion, her husband surprised her with a piano for their home. Hannah says she felt complete now. What once was a void is now filled with joy!

Whenever you feel down or tired, reach in and read it aloud. Smile! And get to work pursuing your passion.

- Visit your local library. Research a new passion. Make a list of what it would entail to pursue. Get started.

- If you've been a collector of something, it might be time to visit the real thing. If you collect miniature hot-air balloons, take a ride on a real one. If you collect colorful toy carousels, visit a carousel museum or go to a park that has one and ride on it. The point is to get up close and personal with your passions.

- So, you really don't think you have any passions? Close your eyes. Take a moment and think about what you most enjoyed doing as a child. Was it bicycling, baking in the kitchen with your mother, drawing, or writing stories? Did you love the beach and water sports, or were you a winter thrill seeker with a love for skiing, sledding, and ice-skating? Were you most fond of strategically competitive games like golf or chess, or did you prefer team sports like soccer and backyard baseball games? For those who are so far removed from their passions and really do not know what they are, this daydreaming exercise is a good starting point to find clues. When you think about the activities you were involved in as a child, you will find clues that might help reveal your passions today.

- Even if you are no longer able to physically play your passion sport, you can find a way to participate in it. If you have a bad knee but miss playing basketball, why not gather the neighbor-hood kids and organize weekly driveway games, or volunteer your time as a coach for inner-city kids who would like to learn the game?

- Maybe you truly never developed a passion. Now's the time to discover one. Ask a coworker about a fun activity she's been talking about at the office or join a friend at her next garden or book club meeting.

CHITCHAT

I often wonder why we, as women, feel guilty wanting our soul food or feel pressure toward giving up our passions. It seems so natural for men to pursue their passions. I watch my husband in amazement. John was once an Ivy League college football star and now collects football memorabilia as a hobby and works as a financial investor for many of his favorite football athletes. He always had a passion for golf and makes it a priority to get on the golf course at least once a week. He always loved the thrill of speed and race cars. He raced dirt bikes when he was fifteen, and now he drags me to car races. He fulfilled his dream of racing last year when he decided to once again act on his passion and enroll in a one-day racing school at Disney World while we were on vacation. What a thrill it was for him, and for me and our two daughters, when we sat in the stands watching his speeding car zip by as the announcer called his name! Now John has found another way to keep his passion alive. He recently bought a small gas-powered remote control model car . . . and "races" every day in the backyard!   —Lisa Lelas

The Key: Attaching This Step to Your Current Lifestyle

· Write your passion somewhere on your to-do list. Set the wheels in motion to get your passion into your life once again. Every day this week, do one thing that can help you get closer to it. Maybe it will mean making a phone call or visiting the library to do research; perhaps it will entail upping your weekly savings a little bit to afford it. Whatever it is, make this week the week for a welcomed change.

- Research your passion on the Internet or at your local library. Create a plan that will lead you closer to your passion.
- Take a class that will instruct, encourage, and enable you to enjoy a new passion.
- If you find your own unique way to attach this step to your personal lifestyle, please share your ideas with us on our Web site: www.SimpleStepsProgram.com.

Sharing

Rediscovering an Old Passion
Brings Kara a New Business
and a New Attitude

Kara is a giver, in every sense of the word. A wife and a mother of three young children, she also runs a small day care service out of her home during the week and spends whatever free time she may have (during naps, evenings, and some weekends) volunteering her time to local charities and civic organizations. She is well respected and admired in her community. Bright, bold, and confident . . . one would think.

After she married, Kara stopped working full-time in the hotel industry. In a flash, nine years went by and she recalls waking up one day and just knowing that something was wrong. "Somewhere along the way, I started losing myself. I lost the Kara in me. The fun-loving, happy Kara. I missed her." She says, "I have twin boys and a little girl. Obviously they need my full attention. But it just seemed as though I did everything for everybody else but me. I went from wearing snazzy suits to wearing stretch pants every day. I gained 60 pounds. It does a number on your psyche. I was the low man on the totem pole in my house. Even my dog came before me!"

What Kara enjoyed most about the ten-week Simple Steps program was that nothing was *taken away* from her. The key was learning moderation and control. "Each week, there were things that were actually *added* to our daily life. We added water, we added vitamins, and we added order to our life, and so on."

When she began the program, Kara recalls, it was like a light went on in her brain. She felt like she had found the inspiration she had been waiting for to make some changes in her life. "It was a fresh start," she said, smiling, and from the very first week on Simple Steps, she knew she was hooked.

Kara applied each Simple Step to her daily lifestyle diligently. She started making better eating choices. In ten weeks she lost 18 pounds, and says she was starting to feel good about herself. "I started taking care of myself," she says. "I even had my hair cut in a beauty salon for the first time in five years. Before, I didn't think I was worth the thirty-five dollars."

It started with small steps, and then Kara took one big step. During week nine on the program, her Simple Steps group began a discussion on passions and the importance of rediscovering lost passions. Right then, Kara felt something tug at her heart. Was this fate staring her right in the eyes, trying to send her a message? She knew she had buried her creative side, her artistic self, years ago. Since she was very young, she had a talent for knitting and sewing and designing. When she came back to her group the very next week, she was excited to report that she had found her old knitting basket collecting dust, and had already purchased a domain name on the Web for her new business. She was excited and ready. Encouraged by the women in her group, she started experimenting with new sweater designs and making original hand-stitched baby blankets out of recycled wool sweaters. As soon as she started showing them, people wanted to buy them. They were entered in a juried art show. Her business was off and running! Many children's boutiques now carry Kara's designs.

Once she started following one passion, she was inspired to do more. "I always thought I could be a good teacher, but I'd never tried it. I now teach knitting. It helps feed my creative side."

Kara weaved her creative side into her volunteer work as well. Working on an exclusive interior designer's show house in town, Kara got to design their Web page and their brochures, and even wrote most of the features that went to the media. She helped design and raise funds for a proposed community playground and was hailed volunteer of the week by a local newspaper. She was even named volunteer of the year by a local civic foundation. She was getting recognition, but most important, Kara was finally filling a creative void inside her soul.

Even though Kara is busier these days, she believes she can give much more of herself now to her family. "I've realized I had to have my own set of passions and goals, and that we all have to keep evolving. I'm evolving again. I don't think that sad person is there anymore. Kara is back!"

Today, Kara still teaches knitting, creates one-of-a-kind baby blankets and sweaters for boutiques, and continues her volunteer work. She is also proud to be a facilitator for the Simple Steps program, now running groups in her hometown.

Congratulations!

You've now mastered the following Simple Steps. Read them aloud
as a positive affirmation. Make them a habit and keep them up as
part of your new lifestyle.

I am drinking eight cups of water daily

I am walking twenty minutes a day

I am clearing out one drawer/cabinet/closet space every week

I am saving $2 a day (or 1 percent of my weekly salary)

I am keeping a daily food journal

I am squeezing in some isometrics every day

I am maintaining an efficient laundry system

I am following a daily to-do list

I am taking a multivitamin every day

I am aware of my posture and breathing

I am keeping a clear desktop

I am cleansing and moisturizing daily

I am replacing bad fats with good fats

I am dancing to at least one song every day

I am maintaining a clean and healthy refrigerator and pantry

I am cleaning and flossing my teeth twice daily

I am cutting back on caffeine

I am discovering the benefits of yoga

I am maintaining a system to avoid mail piles

I am finding daily serenity time

I am replacing processed foods with whole grains

I am doing a few minutes of crunches every day

I am maintaining a clean car

I am dressing smart and keeping my closet organized

I am eating more slowly, respecting food

I am greeting the day with morning stretches

I am organizing my photos

I am keeping a gratitude journal

I am no longer eating at night

I am strength training every week

I am making my bed every morning

I am getting more sleep

I am using herbs and spices daily

I am trying new physical activities each week

I am keeping up with my repair projects

I am rediscovering my passions

The Sunflower

Reaching new heights.
Self-confident and strong.
Magnificent.

Grocery Shopping

Plan Meals Ahead and Set Up an Efficient Grocery Shopping System

Why Should We Set Up an Efficient Shopping System?

- Setting up an efficient shopping system simplifies our life.
- An efficient shopping system is timesaving. We'll spend less time in the grocery store because we'll know exactly what we need and where to find it.
- Setting up an efficient system can save money. Shopping from a grocery list prevents us from buying things that we may already have at home or don't need.
- An efficient shopping system allows us to diversify our meals. When we plan ahead, we can plan to try new recipes instead of the same old thing.
- Learning how to read labels makes us informed shoppers. We make better food choices for our health.
- A shopping list prevents us from making the kind of impulse buys that are bad for our health.
- An efficient system eliminates daily trips to the grocery store.
- Food preparation will lead to healthier at-home snacking with quick-grab produce ready to eat.

- By planning ahead we get control of food. Food no longer controls us.

How to Set Up an Efficient Shopping System

- Organize a weekly meal plan and stick to it. Begin by flipping through cookbooks or your favorite recipe file and choose meals for the upcoming week. Check the Internet; there are many Web sites that have a collection of recipes, such as www.foodtv.com or www.cookinglight.com.
- Plan easy recipes or Crock-Pot meals on your busier days. Or your might want to cook on the weekends and freeze portions for fast weekday meals.
- Try scheduling dinner theme nights to help you incorporate a variety of foods into the week. For example, seafood on Tuesdays and Fridays, different ethnic dishes on Mondays, pasta on Wednesdays, Crock-Pot meals on Thursdays, perhaps a family vote for Saturday's meal, and simple soups, stews, and salads on Sundays. Tailor-make your own schedule according to your family's preferences. Theme nights can make choosing specific recipes easier.
- Add lots of color to your plates. Balance meats with colorful fruits and vegetables. Not only do they look nice on your plate, they have the power to help prevent disease. They contain phytochemicals, plant chemicals that not only give fruits and vegetables their wonderful colors but enhance and protect your health, too.
- Choose meals with protein sources, like chicken, fish, lean meats, and legumes. When considering legumes as your pro-

tein, add whole grains like brown rice; this combination provides amino acids that help build muscle.

- When planning your meals, add fiber-rich whole grains, such
as bulgur, barley, oats, and quinoa, which slowly release their
carbohydrates into your bloodstream, helping your stay alert
and energetic.

- When planning desserts, be smart about sugar. Bake an apple
with cinnamon and nutmeg topped with raisins, or dip your
favorite fruit in a small amount of melted chocolate or yogurt.
Sprinkle chopped mint leaves and toasted coconut over a fresh
fruit salad. (For more suggestions go to www.cookinglight.com.)

- Once you've chosen your recipes, write down all the ingredients
you'll need to make them.

- Most stores have an itemized list of what's contained in each
aisle. Ask for one at the service desk the next time you shop.
Organize your list according to the layout of the store.

- Clip coupons for items on your list. Store coupons in an envelope and write your list on that envelope.

- Make copies of a routine shopping list for your household, or
have an original list stored in your computer of items that you
use each week, such as milk, butter, bread, and cheese. Add
blank lines underneath for jotting down all other food items
needed for that week.

- Now that your pantry is clean, give it a quick weekly inspection
for food items you already have before you go grocery shopping.

- Always build thirty extra minutes into your shopping schedule
to allow time for cleaning, cutting, and preparing food items
immediately upon arriving home from the grocery store.

- As soon as you get home from grocery shopping, cut all visible
fat off of meats and poultry and place them in freezer wrap or
bags. Date the bags/wrap and make sure the air is out of them.

CHATTER TIME

Lucy, a Simple Steps participant and mother of three active teenagers, found a way to finally conquer the daily "What's for dinner?" battle. Every Sunday morning she plans her meals for the upcoming week and posts the list on her refrigerator. Upon reviewing the list, her family has until Sunday evening to request any changes. For example, one week her daughter switched homemade-pizza night to Thursday night when she didn't have soccer practice. The half hour Lucy uses to plan meals on Sunday saves her a week's worth of stress.

- Place a paper towel in with any lettuce you wash and store; it helps absorb water and prevent brown spots.
- Wash all fruits and vegetables (except berries) and place them in see-through containers for easy grabbing.
- Prepare small sandwich bags of fruits and vegetables to take to work or to use as a child's snack.
- Post your weekly meal plan on the refrigerator to remind yourself to pull out any frozen food needed for the next day.
- When making a favorite meal, double the recipe and freeze half. If you do this once a week, you can take one day off from cooking each week. Do this twice a week, and you can have cook-free weekends all month long. Most frozen meals will store safely for up to one month.
- As you test menus, keep a record of your favorites on your computer. The next time you want to make one, you'll have it at your fingertips.

READING LABELS

Nutrition Facts
Serving Size 1 cup (228g)
Servings per Container 2

Amount per Serving
Calories 250   Calories from Fat 110

	% Daily Value*
Total Fat 12g	18%
Saturated Fat 3g	15%
Cholesterol 30 mg	10%
Sodium 470 mg	20%
Total Carbohydrate 31g	10%
Dietary Fiber 0g	0%
Sugars 5g	
Protein 5g	

Vitamin A	4%
Vitamin C	2%
Calcium	20%
Iron	4%

*Percent Daily Values are based on a 2,000 calorie diet. Your Daily Values may be higher or lower depending on your calorie needs:

	Calories:	2,000	2,500
Total Fat	Less than	65g	80g
Sat. Fat	Less than	20g	25g
Cholesterol	Less than	300mg	300mg
Sodium	Less than	2,400mg	2,400mg
Total Carbohydrate		300g	375g
Dietary Fiber		25g	30g

Always make note of the actual serving size and how many servings are in the container.

Note the calories. Remember they are per serving. Notice on this label that almost half of the calories are from fat.

Aim for high-fiber, low-sugar, and low-fat foods.

Levels of vitamins A, C, and D, calcium, and iron are listed on many products, even if they are zero.

Label information is based on a 2,000-calorie diet. Nutritional values will be different for you if your caloric need is higher or lower.

Don't forget to read the ingredients, too. The first three are the primary content. Watch out for hard-to-pronounce words because they are usually chemical fillers.

CHITCHAT

Our mother uses a straw to get the excess air out of her food storage bags that are getting ready to go into the freezer. She fills the bag with a food item and zips up the bag so the straw is the only thing that fits in. Then she sucks out the air in the bag and zips it up. —Linda McClintock and Lisa Lelas

The Key: Attaching This Step to Your Current Lifestyle

- Keep a running list of your frequently used items on your refrigerator so it's handy whenever you go grocery shopping.
- First thing in the morning, clean, cut, and prepare all of your produce for the day (snacks, dinner, etc.).
- While reading the Sunday paper each week, pull out the coupon section and clip any for your favorite food items.
- If you find your own unique way to attach this step to your personal lifestyle, please share your ideas with us on our Web site: www.SimpleStepsProgram.com.

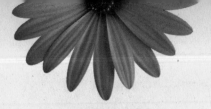

Add More Walking

Extend Your Daily Walk from Twenty to Thirty Minutes

Why Do We Need to Add More Walking?

- We need to change our regular walking routine because our bodies have by now adjusted to our twenty-minute walk, and we may need a new challenge.
- Remember, walking improves circulation and blood levels of mood-boosting hormones. Additional walking will further improve our health.
- As our legs have become stronger and our bodies more efficient over the last nine weeks, we are burning fewer calories when we walk. So we need to walk longer.
- Adding ten minutes to our walk can help break a weight loss plateau. We will burn extra calories and also increase our metabolic rate (the rate at which your body burns calories).
- Increasing our walk by ten minutes can burn as many as 40 additional calories (125 calories in thirty minutes).
- Walking for an additional ten minutes takes us to new places in our neighborhood and forces us to change routes and open our eyes to new things.
- At the end of a stressful day, a walk is still the best way to unwind.

How to Add More Walking

- If time is an issue, split your thirty-minute walk into two fifteen-minute sessions or three ten-minute sessions if necessary.
- The most important thing (besides simply taking your walk) is your pace. Now that you have been walking for nine weeks, it's time to think about walking faster. Remember our explanation of brisk walking from week one? Now, more than ever, you need to increase your pace if weight loss is your desire. *Time your daily walk and thereafter aim to shave a few minutes or even just seconds off your time. As your fitness level increases, your miles covered will increase.*
- Now that you are adding ten minutes, find a new route. We suggest finding a quiet, serene route that appeals to you.
- Now is a good time to add challenges to your walk: speed intervals, hills, walking backward, or perhaps using walking poles.
- Breathe deeply while walking. Breathe in through your nose and expand your belly. Exhale and contract your belly.
- Continue to practice good form. Take short steps, bend and swing your arms, and don't lean forward or backward.
- Add interval training: Walk at a slow pace for two blocks and then speed walk for one block. Repeat throughout the thirty-minute workout. Or you can do intervals in minutes: Walk slowly for two minutes and then speed walk for one minute. Repeat until your workout is complete.

CHITCHAT

My teenage daughter Alicia and I love to walk in the dark. We live in a safe neighborhood and after long hectic days, it's a great way to spend some quality time under the stars. We put on our sneakers and reflective vests, grab the flashlights, and head out. We always have the best conversations during our evening walks together. Alicia and I gab so much that before we know it we're back at our front door. The point is if we were not out walking, Alicia would be in her room listening to music or reading and I would be doing chores around the house. Instead, we are making precious memories while staying healthy together. Grab a family member, and make some memories.

—Beverly Zingarella

The Key: Attaching This Step to Your Current Lifestyle

· Always bring your sneakers when traveling. There may not be a gym around, but there is always somewhere to walk—even if it's in the hotel hallways.

· Buddy up! Once again try to enlist a friend to walk with you first thing in the morning. You will be less likely to skip your morning walk if your partner is waiting at the end of your driveway.

· Take a brisk walk after dinner with your spouse or child. It's a great way to connect on a daily basis and discuss your day.

· Log your walks. Track miles, time, and perhaps how you feel before and after walking. Many Simple Steps ladies keep walking logs and find it motivating to look back and see their progress.

- Challenge the family down the street to a weekly walk-off. Set a time and day to get together and walk around the block. Whichever family finishes first wins. Winners are treated to a family cookout.
- Make a thirty-minute tape of your favorite music. We suggest alternating slow and fast songs to match your speeds.
- Time your daily walks. Challenge yourself to beat your previous time.
- Consider purchasing a pedometer. A pedometer attaches to your clothes and logs how many miles and/or steps you take. Wear it for a few days and calculate your daily average number of steps. Continue to wear the pedometer and change variables such as where you park; take a walk at lunch, take the stairs, and watch your number rise. It's a constant reminder to be more active during the day.
- Join a walking club. If you cannot find a walking club, consider starting your own.
- If you find your own unique way to attach this step to your personal lifestyle, please share your ideas with us on our Web site: www.SimpleStepsProgram.com.

Entryway

Create an Inviting Entryway to Your Home

Why Is It Important to Create an Inviting Entry to Our Home?

- First impressions are important to our guests and to us. The entry to our home is a guest's first impression of us. Creating an inviting entryway gives us a sense of pride when we welcome guests.
- The entry to our home is a direct reflection of our *entire* home. It should feel welcoming and have our personal touches. It establishes the style of the rest of our home.
- We feel more peaceful when we enter a home with a tidy, warm, and inviting entryway.
- Lighting in our entry, in particular, can set the tone for our entire home. Lighting in entryways can enhance our foyer, giving it an inviting feel as well as making it safe.
- Don't allow clutter into your entryway. Scattered shoes, mail, coats, or toys have no place in our entry and can make us feel out of control the minute we walk into our home.
- An organized entryway or foyer makes it easier when we have to

leave our home. If our keys, sunglasses, coat, and shoes are in place, our transition is much quicker and less stressful.

How to Create an Inviting Entryway

- Start outside. Take everything off the front porch or stoop before you begin cleaning. Once the entry is clutter free, sweep the entire area, including stairs and sidewalk. Sweep the doorframe, outside walls, and ceiling for cobwebs.
- Take out any screens and dust or rinse them off. Repair any holes (clear nail polish works) or replace screens if necessary.
- Wash any windows on the door or on your front porch.
- Inspect the hardware on the door, such as doorknob, hinges, and screws. If necessary, tighten or replace hardware.
- If needed, give your front door a fresh coat of paint.
- If the doorbell is not working, replace it.
- Dust and clean lights and replace lightbulbs if necessary.
- Hose off the welcome mat or consider purchasing a new one. Mats can trap 80 percent of household dirt being brought in from outside.
- Wash off cushions from any porch swing or chairs.
- If your mailbox is at your front entryway, paint or replace the box as necessary.
- If you have brick or stone steps or a brick/stone walkway, scrub them down with a mixture of ¼ cup of bleach to 1 gallon of water at least once a year.
- Place flowerpots with colorful flowers on the porch or steps.
- When you think you are done, walk out onto your lawn and approach your entryway. Make sure everything looks neat and tidy. Pull any weeds growing in the walkway. If your entryway is in need of repair and you are unable to do the work yourself,

make a phone call and schedule the repair. Now head inside for more sprucing up.

- Walk in your front door and breathe in. Remember, your home entry reflects you—it should smell fresh and clean. Plug-in air fresheners are available if needed but may not be necessary once you finish this Simple Step.
- Begin cleaning inside by removing everything from your entryway: benches, umbrella stand, coat rack, tables, wall hangings, light fixtures, and whatever else you may have there.
- Dust all wall hangings and clean any glass or mirrors. Clean out the umbrella stand and coat rack.
- Dust the baseboards, ceilings, walls, and corners.
- Thoroughly clean carpet, rugs, or flooring.
- Wash down the walls and the front door, paying close attention to the area near the handle or knob to remove fingerprints or scuff marks.
- Consider whether your foyer could use a fresh coat of paint. Wallpaper, borders, or stencil patterns might create the look you want.
- Once walls, floors, and ceilings are clean, consider your lighting. Replace any lighbulbs that are out.
- Before returning anything to your foyer, look around and assess exactly what you need there. Consider where coats will hang, school/work bags will be stored, and where to put other items you frequently carry into your home. Would a shelf or small table to place mail or groceries on while you hang your coat be convenient? Hang a key rack right next to your entryway for quick grabbing.
- Rehang wall accessories. Mirrors are a great way to give a small foyer a more open feeling.
- Consider hanging family pictures in the foyer for a warm, homey look.

- Exhibit your favorite artwork in your foyer to display your personal style.
- Plants or flowers add an inviting and refreshing feeling to your foyer.
- Every time you return home, be sure to return everything to its proper place, including coats, hats, gloves, keys, etc.

The Key: Attaching This Step to Your Current Lifestyle

- Sweep your porch as part of your weekly cleaning.
- Take five minutes before bed or first thing in the morning and put away anything that does not belong in the foyer.
- Include a monthly foyer organization checklist on your monthly to-do list.
- Make it a habit to buy a bouquet of fresh flowers while grocery shopping every week to place in your foyer.
- If you find your own unique way to attach this step to your personal lifestyle, please share your ideas with us on our Web site: www.SimpleStepsProgram.com.

Treasure Mapping

SIMPLE STEP 40

Create Your Own Treasure Map of Life Goals

Why Should We Create a Treasure Map?

- A treasure map helps turn our dreams into attainable goals. It is a visualization or road map of where we want to go.
- A treasure map is a fun and easy project and creates an artifact that we will cherish throughout our life.
- Our thoughts are energy. *Seeing* our goals, rather than just thinking them, is a much more powerful message to our brain. By changing our thoughts and mental pictures through treasure mapping, we can change our reality.
- Treasure mapping works for us in two ways. It lifts our spirits through *instant gratification*, whereby from the moment we display the treasure map and stare at it, it automatically makes us feel better; we feel good as we glimpse into our fantasy future. Also, it helps us achieve our dreams with *long-term success*. After the novelty of the newly displayed treasure map wears off, our subconscious mind keeps us connected to it and continues to move us closer toward the direction of accomplishing our goals every day.
- Creating a treasure map helps us break through any limitations

we may have set for ourselves. The universe is very giving. Dream big!

How to Create a Treasure Map

· To begin making a treasure map of your dreams and desires, you must have a list of personal goals you wish to accomplish. Be creative; set no limits. Remember, this is for *you* alone, no one else. If you can really imagine yourself doing it or having it, then you can achieve it. Make your list.

CHITCHAT

For as long as I can remember, treasure mapping has been a part of my life. My dad would encourage me as a young girl to list my life's goals on index cards with possible ways to achieve them written beneath each goal. I would cut out visuals to help me clearly see my goals. I watched my parents as European immigrants learn a new language, build a home and family, and start a small business on pure faith. Then I witnessed the tremendous growth of their business over the years. I was in my early twenties before I discovered there was a name for the technique of goal setting I had learned from my parents. Inspirational author Napoleon Hill and other authors referred to it as treasure mapping, and that made sense to me. Mapping out a plan to achieve our desires is indeed like a treasure hunt! After all, with proper planning, our dreams do become a tangible pot of gold!

—Lisa Lelas

- If you feel one goal stands out as something you'd like to achieve quickly, you may design a treasure map with just that specific goal in mind.

- If you are not sure what your goals are at this point, use the next few weeks to determine what they are. Carry around a small goal diary or notebook and list ideas. Look at this list and you will probably find clues there. Remember: Keep your list about *your* goals, not other people's goals for you.

- Once you have your list in place, gather old magazines and sort through them, collecting pictures and phrases that match items you've listed. Feel free to pull out pictures that simply appeal to you, even if they don't correspond directly to any of your goals. Include these images in your treasure map. They might make sense to you at a later time. The amount of goals does not matter. Treasure maps are effective focusing on even just one goal.

- Don't limit yourself. You can seek images that apply to the Simple Steps program for better living or to bigger life goals that might be important to your happiness. You may be experiencing financial hardship after being laid off at work, but that shouldn't stop you from including a picture of a red Ferrari sports car, if that is your desire.

- Get your treasure-mapping supplies together: magazine picture cutouts, poster board (any size), a glue stick, scissors, and a Magic Marker.

- Display your new visual images by adhering them to the poster board in any pattern. Some people divide the display board into equal sections, such as "home and family," "health and fitness," or "career." Some may choose to display their picture cutouts around a photo of themselves or something spiritual. Don't forget to decorate your treasure map with pretty visuals and motivational words and phrases (such as "money" or "I can do it!").

- Hang your treasure map someplace where you will be sure to see it every day. The ideal place would be on your bedroom wall in your line of sight while in bed, or on a wall in your kitchen. If your map includes private dreams, pick a more discreet place such as inside your master closet door or medicine cabinet. The point is you must *see* your treasure map *every day* for it to work.
- It could take days, weeks, months, or longer, but in the end most people find that the opportunities to achieve the goals on their map will appear almost magically.
- Keep an open mind, so that when the opportunity to materialize your dreams arises, you will recognize it and take advantage of it. Use your treasure map to stay positive.

The Key: Attaching This Step to Your Current Lifestyle

- As you flip through magazines, get into the habit of tearing out pictures that seem to move your emotions.
- Start a daily treasure-mapping folder, bin, or basket inside your pantry or on your desk for easy accessibility. Throw in pictures, photos, and ideas after sorting the mail, sorting magazines, or doing any daily de-cluttering.
- Keep a small goal notebook with you throughout the day or jot down goals and dreams in your food journal as you become inspired.
- Begin collecting favorite quotes, inspiring greeting cards, pressed flowers, advertisements, and newspaper headlines. Start seeing your daily life with new eyes. Focus on your future.
- Make your treasure map the size of the inside of your briefcase if you open it throughout the day, or even inside a file folder that opens up, and open it as often as possible.

- Keep your treasure map on the passenger seat of your car if you spend a lot of time running errands or commuting to work.
- Take a digital photo of your treasure map and load it onto your computer as your screen saver.
- Every year or so, as you notice most of your goals have been achieved or as you want to include new ones, update your treasure map. Make a success list of what you have achieved. This should inspire you to create new goals.
- If you find your own unique way to attach this step to your personal lifestyle, please share your ideas with us on our Web site: www.SimpleStepsProgram.com.

Sharing

Kimberly Finds Inspiration
Through Creating a Family
Treasure Map Journal

Call her intuitive, a romantic, or maybe a dreamer. Whatever it is that guides her soul, Kimberly is truly like a sunflower, bright and proud. Family and treasure maps are her water and sun, nourishing her life.

When she joined the Simple Steps program, Kimberly says it was like finding the oxygen mask on a plane. "You put the mask on yourself first. You breathe. Then you put it on your children. You all feel better. You all benefit."

Kimberly is the mother of four teenagers. That's challenging in itself, but she also helps her husband with his equipment company while managing the house. Shuffling the teens around from activity to activity and sometimes working long hours at the office was starting to wear down her energy. "Things get so hectic," she says. "You've really got to simplify and organize and at the same time find a way to be good to yourself. That's where Simple Steps comes in. I just found it to be this miracle in my life."

From the time she was a little girl, Kimberly had always been drawn to pretty things. Simple beauty like rustic birdhouses, a flower-stenciled wall, or images of angels. For as long as she can remember she would cut out magazine pictures of things that appealed to her. She would put them in her wish box and then create colorful collages with them. She didn't realize it then, but she was helping her soul stay connected to her passions. Enthusiasm poured through Kimberly as she sat through week ten of the Simple Steps program and heard that her final assignment (Simple Step #40) was to build a treasure map of her goals and desires. "This is so me!" she thought to herself and couldn't wait to get home to start building.

But this time it was even more. Kimberly was on a magical treasure-mapping life mission, and her family watched in awe of her focus and empowerment. They, too, wanted to be part of the magic. She and her husband began discussing their life dreams. They decided to create a marriage treasure map so they could always keep their goals in sight. It was exciting and a wonderful rebonding experience for both of them. Before long, Kimberly's kids started treasure mapping, too. It seemed to bring the whole family together. Kimberly decided to make a treasure map journal, whereby each page would represent various things dear to her heart, such as her husband, her children, her garden, and her secret wishes, and she included a page for angels.

"These are my ideas and dreams. I feel content when I look at them, my goals for losing weight and my aspirations for my children. It changed my attitude. What's incredible is that I've had many of my wishes come to me without a whole lot of work. I know the power of wishes. I now know the power of treasure mapping. It's as if I visualize what I want, put it in my treasure map journal, and then it comes to me."

Kimberly recalls one recent wish. She had always admired a certain gold link bracelet with a gold heart pendant. "Finally one day I saw it again in a magazine and I cut it out and pasted it into my jour-

292 | WEEK TEN

nal. I never showed it or mentioned it to anyone. Then, on my fortieth birthday, to my amazement, it appeared. My husband had purchased the exact bracelet and he swears he had no idea!"

As she attains one goal, she adds another. There are always new dreams to chase and angels to believe in. Kimberly and her husband dream of having one more child and she's hoping that will be a reality in the near future. But she's taking life one step at a time these days.

Kimberly believes her new outlook on life stems from learning to take time out for herself. "Simple Steps is my soul food nourishing me and everyone in my family."

Congratulations!

You've now mastered the following Simple Steps. Read them aloud as a positive affirmation. Make them a habit and keep them as part of your new lifestyle.

I am drinking eight cups of water daily

I am walking twenty minutes a day

I am clearing out one drawer/cabinet/closet space every week

I am saving $2 a day (or 1 percent of my weekly salary)

I am keeping a daily food journal

I am squeezing in some isometrics every day

I am maintaining an efficient laundry system

I am following a daily to-do list

I am taking a multivitamin every day

I am aware of my posture and breathing

I am keeping a clear desktop

I am cleansing and moisturizing daily

I am replacing bad fats with good fats

I am dancing to at least one song every day

I am maintaining a clean and healthy refrigerator and pantry

I am cleaning and flossing my teeth twice daily

I am cutting back on caffeine

I am discovering the benefits of yoga

I am maintaining a system to avoid mail piles

I am finding daily serenity time

I am replacing processed foods with whole grains

I am doing a few minutes of crunches every day

I am maintaining a clean car

I am dressing smart and keeping my closet organized

I am eating more slowly, respecting food

I am greeting the day with morning stretches

I am organizing my photos

I am keeping a gratitude journal

I am no longer eating at night

I am strength training each week

I am making my bed every morning

I am getting more sleep

I am using herbs and spices daily

I am trying new physical activities each week

I am keeping up with my repair projects

I am rediscovering my passions

I am planning meals and shopping more efficiently

I am walking thirty minutes a day

I am keeping a clean and inviting entryway

I am using a treasure map to attain my goals

THE HARVEST

Reaping
the
Benefits

A Day in the Life of the New You
Health · Weight · Home · Spirit
Putting It All Together

Putting It All Together

A Template for a Healthy Lifestyle

Congratulations! You have completed the Simple Steps lifestyle makeover program. Like a tiny bud transformed into a beautiful flower, your blossom is now open. Your new life awaits you.

We hope that we may have helped you peek into the silver lining of your soul, that you feel better, perhaps more energetic, less stressed, or simply more positive; that you have gotten some control over clutter and you lead a more organized, productive life; and that you may have picked up a few good habits to take with you on your life's journey.

You should not feel overwhelmed at the thought of practicing all forty steps every day. On the following pages we have included simple guidelines and tips toward maintaining all the steps on a regular basis quite effortlessly. What you take out of the program is totally up to you. You might find yourself more drawn to one particular area that needs your attention, such as home or diet. Now that your life (diet, exercise, home, and self) are in basic order because you've completed the ten-week program, it's time for you to figure out where you want to go next. A good place to start is to ask yourself, which aspect of the Simple Steps program was most rewarding for me?

Maybe you're glad your house is in better order now, but what has really transformed your life turned out to be the exercise. Well, now you know that your next goals should focus on exercise and how you can make it a bigger part of your everyday life.

Or maybe you're glad you finally lost those 10 pounds, but what has really made you happier is the fact that your house is more orderly. The next set of goals you focus on should obviously have to do with your home. Do you want to redecorate? Or renovate? Take on a bigger organization project, like your basement or attic? Maybe even start a business organizing and redecorating for others?

The point is once you recognize what you enjoy most, you can follow your passion and dreams anywhere.

Diet, Fitness, Home, Self

Forty Steps to a New You!

Here are some tips for easily putting them all together on a regular basis (believe it or not, we have tied all forty Simple Steps into these seven tips).

- **Be honest with yourself.** Being truthful and knowledgeable about the food you eat is the key to unlocking the door to your healthy living. Start at the beginning. A clean refrigerator and pantry and a smart shopping list ultimately give you a healthy base. Flavor your life with nutty whole grains, low-fat recipes seasoned with pungent herbs and spices, and crunchy fruits and vegetables. Savor each bite of your new healthy life.
- **Map out a daily exercise hour.** Upon finishing the program, you should organize everything you've learned about fitness and plan one hour each day for your exercise routine, even if you have to split it up into segments. For example, stretch for a couple of minutes every morning before you start your thirty-minute walk. Plan your strength training for twice a week, and cross-train, do yoga, and dance on the other days. Begin or end each exercise session with a few minutes of abdominal crunches. And if you throw in your isometrics at various mo-

ments throughout your day, it will be easy to put together an hour of exercising each day without becoming overwhelmed or bored with it.

- **Develop a place for everything and put everything in its place.** Ready, set, now *stay* organized! A pristine home is like a beautiful painting. It must begin with a clean palette. Toss the clutter. It simply makes all your organizational projects so much easier. Making your bed and sorting the mail is a daily chore and doing your laundry a weekly chore, but you can also maintain an orderly home without a lot of extra daily effort. Even just an hour or so a week can keep your drawers and closets straightened out, your desktop clear, and your car clean. Be creative. Reserve time on your calendar for things like organizing photos, home fix-it projects, or redecorating.

- **Treat yourself to a little pampering every day.** Let's face it— when we leave our home in the morning feeling good about ourselves, we always seem to have a great day. It's that "good-hair day" thing. When we dress smart and comfortable with our skin clean and glowing, hair in place, and teeth sparkling, we radiate confidence. Make these simple pamper-me rituals a part of your daily routine.

- **Purchase a blank journal.** With this one item you will be able to maintain several important steps. Keep your journal always open on your countertop or carry it with you throughout the day. On the top of the left page, keep a daily log of the food you eat and the glasses of water you drink. Don't forget to check off your vitamins. Use the bottom of that page to write your gratitude entries. On the right page, keep your daily to-do list. You can also keep a cumulative list of future goals and passions boxed in at the bottom.

- **Balance your checkbook and open up a savings account.** Con-

tinue nurturing your $2-a-day savings (or 1 percent of your
weekly salary) and watch the money tree grow!

· **Surrender to serenity.** You can't fight it anymore. Daily calm
time leads to a balanced life with renewed energy. Limiting
your caffeine intake helps ease you into serenity modes and
allows you a more restful sleep. And by not eating at night, you
allow your body to take a break and rejuvenate its systems.

You have so much to feel grateful for. You have completed ten
weeks of self-nurturing, and that in itself is an accomplishment for
most of us. Move forward. Keep your passions alive and think positive. Stay true to your heart, and always try to see your very best reflection. You have, indeed, become a sunflower . . . now capable of
reaching amazing new heights.

We'd love to hear from you. Please check into our Web site,
www.SimpleStepsProgram.com, and give us feedback. We have developed a wonderful network for Simple Steps participants everywhere!

Enjoy your Simple Steps journey, always!

Lisa, Linda, and Beverly

The authors would like to hear from you. If you are interested in putting together a Simple Steps workshop in your community, please write, enclosing a #10 self-addressed stamped envelope to:

Simple Steps Program
c/o Reflections Lifestyle Makeover Workshops
P.O. Box 128
Guilford, CT 06437

The authors are available for lectures and workshops based upon this book. Details will be sent upon request.

Questions or comments can be sent via E-mail:
SimpleStepsProgram@hotmail.com

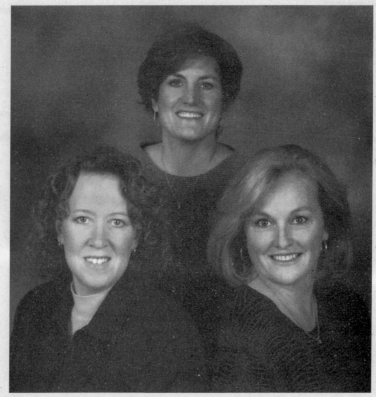

Lisa Lelas (right) is a personal life coach, motivational speaker, and newspaper columnist ("Life Styling"). A former New York City casting director, she is now married and has two young daughters. **Linda McClintock** (center) is a corporate recruiter turned stay-at-home mom with a background in nutrition and healthy gourmet cooking. **Beverly Zingarella** (left) is a stay-at-home mother of three children. Collectively known as the "Guilford Girls" (after their home base of Guilford, Connecticut), they have appeared several times on *Oprah*.